Pain
control

Pain Control

Norman Trieger, D.M.D., M.D.

Professor and Chairman,
Department of Dentistry, Oral and Maxillofacial Surgery,
Montefiore Medical Center and Albert Einstein College of
Medicine, Bronx, New York;
Formerly Professor and Chairman of Oral Surgery,
University of California, Los Angeles

SECOND EDITION

with 71 illustrations

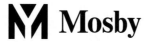 Mosby

St. Louis Baltimore Boston Chicago London Madrid Philadelphia Sydney Toronto

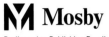

Mosby

Dedicated to Publishing Excellence

Editor-in-Chief: Don Ladig
Executive Editor: Linda L. Duncan
Developmental Editor: Melba Steube
Project Manager: Mark Spann
Production Editor: Stephen C. Hetager
Manuscript Editor: Rhadika Rao Gupta
Layout Artist: Kathy Wiegand
Manufacturing Supervisor: Betty Richmond
Designer: David Zielinski

SECOND EDITION

Printed in the United States of America

Mosby–Year Book, Inc.
11830 Westline Industrial Drive
St. Louis, Missouri 63146

ISBN 1-55664-284-9

94 95 96 97 98 CA/MV 9 8 7 6 5 4 3 2 1

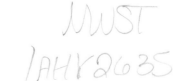

This book is dedicated
to my teachers and my students.

Preface

The preface to the first edition was written over 20 years ago. Since that time there have been a series of remarkable advances that profoundly affect the management of pain and anxiety. We have seen basic changes in our understanding of the biology of the nervous system. Neurotransmitters, neuromodulators, and receptor agonist and antagonist behaviors are better understood, and dramatic new methods of measuring and monitoring a patient's physiologic responses have evolved. New drugs such as midazolam are rapidly displacing diazepam; propofol may replace methohexital, and new potent opioids have been introduced along with specific antagonists to cause reversal of effects.

State practice laws have changed to now require special licensure for dentists using sedation or general anesthesia. Intravenous medications have been more widely used for a variety of endoscopic procedures and minor office surgeries by several different subspecialties in medicine. Mortality and significant morbidity have fortunately declined appreciably.

The guiding principles of this book remain true to the tenets of the original edition: individual patient evaluation; management leading to careful titration of medications; fitting the method to the patient and not the patient to the method.

The updating of this book has been an exciting labor—one which will be rewarding to the reader.

Norman Trieger

Contents

Pain
control

1

The Spectrum of Pain Control Today

Dentistry is changing: dental technology, concepts of disease, and methods of improved patient management have advanced steadily over the past century, with a marked quickening of their pace in the last four decades. Basic biologic research advances, along with a change in the cultural values of our society, are to be credited for these improvements. Pain, suffering, and disease have often been interpreted as a punishment for misdeeds or a divine trial. Many of these primitive ideas yielded to the enlightenment that followed scientific discoveries of the etiology of illness—of pathogenic bacteria, fungi, and viruses. Further basic research has begun to clarify the role of autoimmune mechanisms, toxins, and developmental and hereditary abnormalities in the genesis of disease and human suffering. Yet a more sophisticated form of these primitive beliefs still exists in many places, even in modern civilized societies.

Not too long ago, and still fresh in the memories of people now living, surgical procedures in dentistry were performed without benefit of any pain-relieving agents. After all, local anesthesia is a child of this century, and it took many years of education, after its introduction, to achieve a modicum of regular use for the suffering patient. But apart from the ready availability of anesthetics, and improved education on the use of the techniques required, stands the old problem of primitive and punitive attitudes. Some practitioners still believe they are working on unattached teeth and betray their callousness to patients by insisting on inflicting pain and discomfort in the guise of beneficial treatment.

There are many uncomfortable procedures satisfactorily performed regularly in the dental office with the doctor and his or her staff offering only emotional support and which the patient tolerates quite well with this strong bond of rapport. This interaction between doctor and patient is the basis of all therapeutic efforts. Successful practitioners learn to develop a chairside manner in dealing with patients that is of mutual benefit. Despite the many psychologic deterrents to regular dental care, a knowledgeable and empathetic doctor can still effectively treat many patients. But there are, unfortunately, even more patients who are unavailable for regular care because of significant emotional barriers. These patients often require pharmacologic help to facilitate or overcome their fears and anxieties.

There is presently available to every dentist a wide spectrum of psychologic and pharmacologic methods and materials to control pain and anxiety in the dental office. Graphically depicted (Fig. 1-1), the spectrum represents a continuum of patient management. One of the basic concepts of this book is that *every patient, based on individual needs and past history, can be carried successfully through dental treatment.* Dentists and dental schools must educate themselves and their patients to understand this broadened spectrum rather than think in terms of only "local" or "general" anesthesia.

Added to the primary concept of a broad approach to pain control and patient management is the second basic concept: *individualization.* Each patient, a unique person with specific needs for appropriate management, refutes the

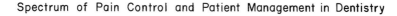

Spectrum of Pain Control and Patient Management in Dentistry

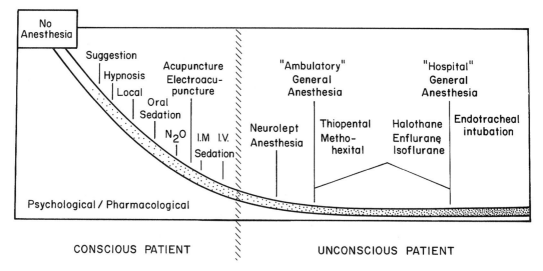

Fig. 1-1. Dentistry is practiced with the aid of a wide spectrum of adjuncts to help overcome anxiety and pain. These include techniques for the conscious patient as well as general anesthesia. Each patient can be individually evaluated and treatment can be modified to satisfy his or her need.

idea of the "average dose" of medication. Collectively, we can be described by a bell-shaped curve of dose/response (Fig. 1-2). Pharmacologists and physiologists rely on this distribution curve to indicate that the majority of people will respond to a particular agent at a particular dosage. But there is always a significant number of persons who are extraordinarily sensitive or inordinately resistant. When dealing with individual patients it is imperative to consider the uniqueness of each patient and anticipate the dose/response.

Psychologic Methods of Pain Control

Pain perception, being a complex bio-psychosocial phenomenon, may be influenced and altered by variety of nonpharmacologic approaches. Anxiety and fear of dental manipulation and treatment significantly influence the quest for dental care as well as the response to therapy. It has been found that more than 10% to 15% of adults are highly fearful and avoid routine dental care while a smaller percentage are overtly phobic to the point of avoiding even emergency visits.[1,2] Psychologic techniques in-

volving cognitive behavior modification may substantially change the patient's thinking, feeling, and behavior. One of the key methods, in addition to providing unambiguous and less threatening information, is to allow the patient the perception of increased control over stimulus events. Learning relaxation, imagery, hypnosis, and the use of various techniques such as acupuncture, acupressure, and transcutaneous electrical stimulation in addition to supportive measures during the treatments are all variably effective in patient management (Chapter 2 contains an expanded discussion).

Adjuncts to Psychologic Management

There are some patients who will resist any suggestion that they need premedication. There are even some patients who regularly refuse local anesthesia, insisting that they dislike the numbing effects of the regional anesthetic block, particularly if it lingers past the appointment period. The use of oral sedative drugs prior to a dental visit is often helpful but is fraught with difficulties such as guessing the amount required for effectiveness.

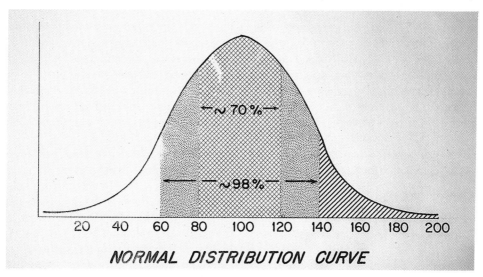

NORMAL DISTRIBUTION CURVE

Fig. 1-2. For a given dose of medication to a large population, approximately 91% will respond within two standard deviations of the mean. Some persons will be extraordinarily sensitive and some will be inordinately resistant.

Effectiveness depends on many factors, including individual susceptibility to the agent, the patient's level of excitement and apprehension, and whether the drug is rapidly or slowly absorbed from the stomach, etc. At best, giving an oral sedative to a patient about to undergo a dental procedure serves primarily as a message to that patient: "I am concerned about your comfort and understand your apprehension." Such a message helps to establish rapport, improves the overall relationship, and makes work easier for both the patient and the dentist. Benzodiazepine medication such as triazolam (Halcion) has been recently shown to have helpful anxiolytic effects in dental surgery.[3]

Nitrous Oxide Sedation

The resurgence of interest in nitrous oxide–oxygen sedation has been remarkable. It has produced a new generation of enthusiastic adherents. Properly administered, it seeks to provide sedation that is free of excitement and hypoxia. Once some patients have experienced nitrous sedation, they insist upon it for any further dental treatment. Others are intolerant to the point of tearing off the nose piece when they begin to feel the characteristic alterations of sensation.

Recent studies have raised the specter of low-dose, long-term exposure to nitrous oxide causing deleterious effects.[4] A mail survey of more than 30,000 dentists and more than 30,000 dental assistants indicated increased health problems and reproductive difficulties in those occupationally exposed to nitrous oxide. In particular, liver, kidney, and neurologic diseases showed significant increases, and among female assistants the incidence of spontaneous abortion was also significantly increased. Emphasis has been placed on the need to reduce office pollution of nitrous oxide gas by better controls of administration and improved methods of evacuating waste gas.

Acupuncture

The insertion and stimulation of acupuncture needles in animals and in humans has been shown to cause the release of endogenous endorphins with a consequent analgesic effect of varying degree. This effect can be blocked by pretreatment with the narcotic antagonist naloxone hydrochloride. Although the technique of acupuncture does not enjoy wide usage in modern dental practice, it does have application in certain patients with chronic pain and has been a helpful research tool in our understanding of the mechanisms of pain perception.

Transcutaneous nerve stimulation often produces similar analgesic effects and is more widely used for relief of localized chronic pain.

Intramuscular Sedation

Intramuscular sedation, used routinely before general anesthesia in the hospital, has also been used to premedicate children and adults prior to office procedures. There is greater reliability of absorption, but effectiveness still depends on individual variability and the level of initial excitement. Often, a child premedicated to the point of somnolence will awaken and resist manipulative procedures, slipping back into somnolence again when the stress of the operation is over. Depression of respiration caused by such deep level of sedation requires caution and specific preparation by the doctor should it become necessary to assist respiration until the effects of the drugs have worn off.

Intravenous Sedation

The most accurate and effective premedication for the conscious patient is that achieved by gradually titrating a sedative drug directly into a vein. The response is quickly discerned. A variety of agents have been successfully used to lessen the patient's anxiety and have made local anesthesia more effective. The goal is to produce a light level of sedation and avoid central nervous system depression. The patient should remain awake, cooperative, and entirely responsive to direction.

General Anesthesia (Unconsciousness)

The spectrum of pain control includes the management of the unconscious patient. There are large numbers of people who have been successfully, safely, and inexpensively treated in oral surgery offices while under "ambulatory" general anesthesia. Many patients insist on be-

ing totally unconscious for their dental and surgical care. Such care requires that the doctor have extensive education and training, for he or she must be knowledgeable and properly prepared and equipped. The management of an individual who has lost his or her protective reflexes depends on the anesthetist's ability to ensure safety and survival.

Preanesthetic evaluation of patients is often the key to proper management. When evaluation indicates a significant impairment of cardiopulmonary status, the patient should be referred for hospitalization and further consultation. Hospital general anesthesia is reserved for higher risk patients and for those requiring extensive dental and oral surgical care in the hospital operating room. Such hospital management often makes use of an endotracheal tube to ensure an adequate and controlled airway for the delivery of inhalation anesthetics often used in conjunction with intravenous hypnotics. Postoperative care becomes the responsibility of highly trained recovery room personnel.

The spectrum of available approaches to patient management has been described. Each of the "signposts" identified in Fig. 1-1 will be explored in depth in succeeding chapters.

Education for Pain Control

A number of years ago a small group of dentists wisely pointed to a rather large sampling of patients who were not amenable to routine dental treatment. These patients were handicapped, in some instances by physical and mental retardation. A surprisingly larger number of other patients are handicapped by the fear and apprehension of dental procedures. Although the immediate reaction to such problem patients often was varying degrees of derision for their "cowardice," compassionate and empathetic professionals sought to ameliorate the emotional block by offering psychologic and pharmacologic adjuncts. Early pioneers in pain and anxiety control such as the Monheims and the Jorgensens persisted. Through their efforts and the efforts of many more dedicated dentists and teachers, the practice of dentistry and the management of the dental patient has undergone significant changes.

In a recent poll sponsored by the American Dental Society of Anesthesiology and the American Dental Association, it was noted that more than 30% of practicing dentists now use adjunctive agents in addition to local anesthesia. Many dentists have secured advanced education in anesthesiology and practice various techniques of pain control, sedation, and general anesthesia to provide more effective dental treatment for more people. In the past, objections and adverse reactions to these dentists using advanced methods of pain control came not so much from the medical profession but rather from misinformed dentists. What has been recognized and endorsed in recent yeares is that pain and anxiety control, in all of its manifestations, *is* an integral part of the practice of dentistry.

There is a clear-cut distinction to be made between the conscious and the unconscious patient. The "Guidelines on the Teaching of Pain and Anxiety Control" adopted by the American Dental Association's House of Delegates in October 1971 offer a valid explanation by saying, *"the conscious patient is defined as one with intact protective reflexes, including the ability to maintain an airway, and who is capable of rational response to question or command."*[5] There is an impressive variety of agents and techniques that provide for control of pain, anxiety, and apprehension while maintaining a conscious patient—one more cooperative and amenable to dental treatment.

Many dental practitioners have rendered excellent service to their patients through the years and have never used more than local anesthesia supplemented by a mutually satisfactory doctor-patient relationship. Generally, these practices are the result of a selective *distillation* of patients so that those who accept such treatment are helped and reassured. These doctors have made and will continue to make their contribution to the oral health of their patients. The impetus for them to use anything in addition to local anesthesia is minimal and their motivation for advanced or continuing education in the area of pain control will also be minimal.

CONTINUING AND POSTGRADUATE EDUCATION

On the other hand, many of the graduates of dental schools who, over the past 25 or so years, have been building their practices, have found a distinct need for *something* to aid in the management of their patients so that they can fulfill their dental responsibilities. This has led to the great resurgence of interest in nitrous oxide-oxygen sedation. Most dentists who have become interested in nitrous oxide have made determined efforts to secure advanced education and training in its use. The major thrust for these educational courses came *not* from the schools but from state and local societies and independent continuing education programs in a few universities. Schools generally have been predominantly preoccupied with undergraduate and graduate education and have provided only a modicum of instruction for continuing education.

Since the educational guidelines were approved by the American Dental Association, many more schools are offering courses in "Comprehensive Pain and Anxiety Control" to their undergraduate students. The guidelines wisely prescribed that continuing education courses in pain control (1) be limited to the management of the *conscious patient,* (2) provide for didactic *and* clinical experience within a school, hospital, or similar institution, and (3) be designed to ensure *at least* the equivalent of similar courses given to undergraduate students.[5]

Many school clinics and all hospitals maintain year-round service to patients. Many graduate dentists will eagerly avail themselves of the opportunity to spend a limited period (e.g., 1 month) in an active treatment center to learn the essentials of patient care and the limitations of the various methods in use. It may not be too farfetched to consider providing opportunities for continuing education courses during hours when clinics are normally closed. In many large municipal hospitals, operating rooms are now scheduling less emergent cases in addition to emergencies well past the usual closing time in order to keep pace with the increased demand

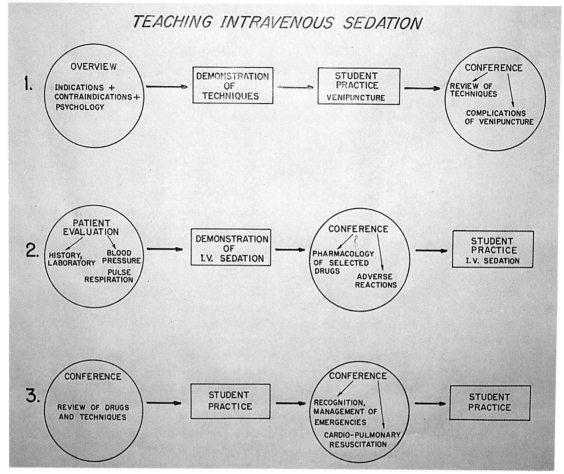

Fig. 1-3. Small groups, several instructors, and supervised clinical participation, presented together with the necessary didactic information, leads to highly motivated and knowledgeable students.

for operating time and to counteract the enormous costs of such expensive facilities standing idle. School and hospital dental clinics may well become centers of active patient treatment and professional education after 5:00 P.M. The demand for patient care is increasing and so is the demand for teaching facilities and faculty.

COURSE STRUCTURE AND CONTENT

Educators favor courses that do not presume to teach everything in a 2-or 3-day composite. We learn in small increments and require reinforcement and experience to achieve meaningful in-

tegration of information. Learning also involves a considerable amount of selective listening—the lecture method is a poor teaching device, especially when one is teaching material that involves, to a considerable extent, manipulative skills, observation, trial, and retrial.

My experience with teaching intravenous sedation courses has shown that if students first overcame the "psychologic skin barrier" and were successful in starting a saline infusion, they became much more receptive to subsequent important information about the drugs and patient reactions. Until students had tried and successfully performed a venipuncture, they maintained a mental reservation as to whether or not they could *use* the rest of the information. Small groups, several instructors, short presentations of didactic material followed by demonstrations, then by participation, produced a highly motivated and knowledgeable student (Fig. 1-3).

What should be the course content? It becomes obvious that the curriculum for a continuing education course should be selective. Although there is a great diversity of pharmacologic agents used to effect sedation and tranquilization, the course should focus on a very limited number in order to develop greater insight into their actions, side effects, etc.

The course must include material relevant to the careful evaluation of each individual patient. Information about applied pulmonary and cardiovascular physiology can and should be integrated with its pertinence to the medical history and evaluation. The pharmacologic effects must also be related to any underlying medical condition rather than be discussed in a nonclinically oriented pharmacology lecture. A realistic assessment of potential hazards is always in order but is often overdone. An essential component of all courses on pain control should be a comprehensive review of the recognition and management of complications and emergencies.

Whenever possible, aspects of technique should actually precede the didactic presentations or at least be briefly presented and then reinforced after the technique has been experienced. The information will then have greater significance and pertinence.

Several follow-up studies of such courses[6,7] have shown that almost 60% of the doctors attending the courses initiated the use of intravenous techniques for conscious sedation in their private offices without any significant incidence of morbidity or mortality.

Comprehensive pain control courses for conscious patient care in continuing education should be at least 60 instructional hours in length, of which one third to one half is spent in clinically supervised training. This program should include pertinent didactic basic sciences and the recognition and management of emergencies and resuscitation. By learning the wider spectrum of agents and methods available, the practitioner will avoid the abuse of any one modality. No one method is applicable to all patients, and individualization for each patient's needs will be the hallmark of competence.

PROFESSIONAL SCHOOL UNDERGRADUATE EDUCATION

Many dental schools are undergoing major curriculum revisions. Emphasis is being slowly shifted to condensing required courses and instituting electives that coincide with the individual's interest and aptitude. Many schools will find the opportunity to provide clinical electives in pain control and patient management beyond the essentials taught in the early undergraduate years.

Teaching the basic sciences of anatomy, physiology, biochemistry, and pharmacology is a significant part of the undergraduate curriculum—students often do not know precisely why they had to learn "all that stuff." In considering the medical evaluation and management of a dental patient about to receive some adjunctive drugs one finds the real "raison d'etre" for the study of basic sciences. *Treating a patient and not a tooth, or treating the whole patient and not an isolated dental disease does require specific knowledge of that individual.* The teaching of pain control and conscious patient management provides a converging point for the basic and clinical sciences.

It is certainly not enough to teach the mechanics of inhalation or intravenous sedation; it is important that they be integrated with the didactic material. Most of the basic sciences taught in dental schools can be meaningfully integrated into the learning of "Patient Management." These courses may be better taught by several teachers with varying backgrounds and selected inputs. For example, a member of the hospital's anesthesiology department, a pharmacologist, a knowledgeable internist, a psychologist, etc., may all contribute their expertise. It would be equally important to have a well-trained and experienced dentist direct or coordinate the program and provide the special insights into dental office patient management.

POSTPROFESSIONAL SCHOOL GRADUATE EDUCATION

General anesthesia requires advanced education and training, which is usually taken for at least 1 year in the department of anesthesiology of a hospital. Recently, 2-year residency programs have developed in cooperation with Departments of Dentistry and Anesthesiology. Graduate students spend all their time in the general operating rooms and in the outpatient clinic of the dental department learning all phases of anesthesiology practice and theory. This background prepares them for an in-depth understanding of the management of patients who require total unconsciousness for their dental care. The dental treatment of physically, neurologically, and emotionally handicapped patients is made possible by the use of general anesthesia.

Summary

Modern dental practice utilizes a broad spectrum of approaches to control pain and anxiety. The dentist should think in terms of the wide variety of psychologic and pharmacologic adjuncts to treatment. The former concept of either "local or general anesthesia" has given way to several methods of accomplishing sedation and cooperation in the conscious patient: these include suggestion, hypnosis, acupuncture, electroacupuncture, local anesthesia, and oral, intramuscular, and intravenous premedication. The treatment of the unconscious patient including the deeply sedated patient is limited to practitioners who have had advanced education and training in general anesthesiology.

The overall aim is to *individualize* patient care by providing the most appropriate method of pain and anxiety control for that person: to fit the method to the patient, not the patient to the method.

References

1. Dworkin SF: Psychological considerations for facilitating anesthesia, and sedation in dentistry. NIH Consensus Conference, Bethesda, Md, April 1985.
2. Friedman N. *Psychosedation. Part 2: Iatrosedation.* In McCarthy, editor: *Emergencies in dental practice—prevention and treatment,* ed 3, Philadelphia, 1979, WB Saunders.
3. Dionne R, Hargreaves K, Kaufman E: Effectiveness of oral triazolam in relieving patient anxiety during outpatient surgery, *Newsletter (AADR & IADR) Res Digest* 4:3, 1990.
4. Eger EI: *Nitrous oxide/N$_2$0,* New York, 1985, Elsevier.
5. American Dental Association, Council on Dental Education: *Guidelines for pain and anxiety control,* Chicago, 1982, American Dental Association, p 152.
6. Trieger N. Teaching intravenous sedation: follow-up of 200 dentists, *Anesth Prog* 25:154-156, 1978.
7. Malamed SF: Continuing education in intravenous sedation; survey of 188 dentists, *Anesth Prog* 28:33-36, 1981.

2

The Significance of Pain in Dentistry

Pain hurts! The amelioration of pain can be accomplished by a variety of techniques that affect the psychologic as well as the physical components of pain perception. Examples of the interrelationship between these two components are numerous. Laboratory experiments of human pain never quite replicate studies of clinical pain. Many variables influence pain perception while the absolute thresholds remain fairly constant.[1]

Cultural and ethnic influences modify the experience of pain[2], and Melzack and Scott[3] have shown that early life experiences affect the perception of pain. In one of their revealing experiments they reared litter mate puppies in two different environments, one normal and the other with sensory deprivation. Dogs raised in the normal environment quickly learned to avoid pain-causing stimuli whereas those raised in the sensory-deprived situation repeatedly burned their noses on the flame of a match and made no move to avoid a needle pricking their skin. They did, however, flinch and make reflex twitches to the stimuli, indicating that they "felt something" but that their integration of the stimuli into a meaningful pain response was lacking. This would indicate that learning plays a primary role in pain response.

Management of Children

The management of children undergoing dental treatment deserves special consideration, particularly with regard to their psychologic growth and well-being. The idea that childhood is a time of pure bliss to which we all look backward with longing is tarnished when we recall the many anxieties that children face. Many of these fearful situations present problems that the child must conquer in order to develop normal controls and resilience. No child can or should be protected from all of them, and it would be impossible to remove all the anxiety from dental procedures. However, we can be clearly aware of the terror present under a relatively calm exterior. We should avoid unnecessarily frightening children and help them develop a better attitude toward future dental and medical care for themselves and, later, their own families. Parents who have pleasant recollections of proper preparation are likely to be useful both to the dentist and to their children at such a time.

The most fundamental response to be assimilated under these circumstances is anxiety. A universal emotion, it is generally much greater in children. Anxiety involves a state of heightened tension with the apprehension and expectation of some harm about to occur. Children may manifest anxiety by becoming tremulous and silent, with rapid, shallow breathing, dilated pupils, and inhibition of most movements. Or they may show hyperactivity with shouting, combativeness, and forceful negativism. However, the underlying dread and expectation of harm are present in both types of reaction. Children's understanding of what is happening and the special childhood fantasies about being hurt, overwhelmed, or crushed combine to magnify the terror. With their inability to understand goes a surprising amount of distortion and confusion about what is being done and about the advice and information that they have been given by others.

9

Children have many reasons for bringing their special worries and concerns to the treatment situation, especially when deprived of parental support. They are confronted with strange instruments; there is the physical insecurity of the "seat on high", without much support, in an unusual kind of chair; and there is the approach to their organs of *speech, eating,* and *defense.* The work of Jessner, Blom, and Waldfogel on reactions of children to tonsillectomy has shown both immediate and subsequent effects.[4] In younger children, fears of separation, abandonment, and mutilation seemed to come up without regard to the objective dangers involved. Some children showed concerns about losing parts of the body, and there were some conceptions of anesthesia as a threat of death. It is important to emphasize that these were unselected children and were not studied for their emotional problems but as average youngsters. In older children the threat of a general anesthetic caused a fear of loss of control. These children were studied following their tonsillectomies and showed a variety of nightmares, fears, sleep disturbances, bed-wetting, and other signs of severe emotional tension at home, symptoms that generally tended to abate after several weeks.

Thus, a procedure that traditionally has been considered quite benign produced marked fears and reactions in children. It took a fairly long time for the anxieties to become assimilated. This does not mean that such procedures are damaging to the child's development; rather, it indicates that they constitute a major stress and that their "traumatic" potentials should not be ignored. Baldwin's studies of stress in children undergoing dental extractions indicated that these are highly stressful events, capable of producing measurable physiologic and psychologic responses.[5]

The parent should be present in the examining room with the child. The dentist must remain in charge of the situation and not permit the parent to subvert the procedure by hovering about and persistently inquiring if the child is being hurt. The dentist may have to direct the parent's behavior at the outset, even before he

or she can gain the child's confidence. In most cases the presence of the parent, albeit an anxious one, is of major help because it helps to quell the child's fear of separation. It also has a salutary effect on the parent, who does not feel immediately shut out by being separated from the child. Confronting the parent with the reality of what is being done diminishes some of the more desperate images he or she may have of the child being hurt or terrified. It is preferable for the parent to enter the treatment room and take part in the induction of anesthesia. Confident suggestions by parent and dentist that the child will behave well will often result in cooperative behavior.

Honesty and deliberate actions are essential in dealing with youngsters. Children should never be tricked, deceived, or told that something is painless when it isn't so. False mannerisms and "cuteness" on the part of the operator will only alarm the child. People who do not like to work with children "telegraph" their feelings, producing a vicious cycle in which they continue to feed ever-increasing amounts of negativeness into the situation. Almost everyone talks to children in a somewhat different tone of voice, and this is fine, so long as it is not overdone.

Plans of treatment should not be discussed with the parent as if the child were not present. The child may understand and be frightened, or he or she may not comprehend and become even more upset. Older children (7 to 12 years of age) need adequate opportunity to verbalize some of their concerns about what is going to happen. An appropriate appeal to their adultlike capabilities has distinct advantages. Whenever possible, appointments should be arranged with an active acknowledgement of their other scheduled activities. Whenever the child can be enlisted to cooperate in the procedure this should be encouraged over forcing, although this cannot always be arranged.

Frequently, because of the emergency nature of a problem, the dentist must set up and perform the necessary treatment within a few minutes. This is not the time to explore the child's fantasy world but to explain what must be done as succinctly and clearly as possible. With a firm approach, but one that will not intensify the child's alarm, the dentist may carry the task to completion despite the protestations of the youngster. Once the treatment is finished, the child may realistically evaluate the facts and see that he or she has been helped, not duped or damaged.

Local anesthesia used in conjunction with other sedation is preferable for most older children, particularly when the operative procedure is limited to one or two areas of the mouth. This enables the child to cooperate and avoids some of the fears and apprehension inherent in the use of a general anesthetic. The momentary pain of a needle prick is well tolerated if it is expected by the child. The dentist should tell the child directly what is about to happen, explaining that it will "pinch" for just a moment and then will not hurt afterward. This is reassuring in the long run and leads to a better acceptance of the dentist. The fundamental job is not to avoid all pain for the child but to get across the purpose of the work and make absolutely clear that the dentist is standing by and forthrightly doing the job of helping.[6]

Adult Anxiety and Pain

In adults, studies have shown the significant role of anxiety in the perception of pain. Beecher's[7] now-classic study of pain in wounded soldiers during World War II demonstrated a remarkable difference in the request for pain medication between these soldiers who had survived warfare and now had their "ticket home" and a comparable civilian population following injury: 32% for military and 83% for civilian patients.[8,9] Egbert carried these studies further to show that patients requests for postoperative pain medication could be reduced by more than one half if the anesthesiologist visited the patient and provided realistic preoperative information and empathetic concern.[10,11]

It is important to realistically advise an oral surgical patient during the consultation visit about the postoperative course, including when and for how long pain may be anticipated. This is repeated when postoperative instructions are given. Specifically, postoperative pain may be severe for 8 to 12 hours after the local anesthetic wears off, and the patient is provided pain medication for this period. Patients are further advised that by the following day their pain will abate, though they should expect soreness that will respond to mild analgesics.

In a high percentage of cases, patients returning the following week report this exact sequence. They are thus provided with a program and know what to expect, which serves to lessen anxiety. The doctor's home telephone number can be provided in the event a weekend or holiday recess follows surgery. (In almost 35 years of a surgical practice, only a small handful of patients called this author—in some cases they were checking to be reassured and did not request the doctor to see them until the day the office was regularly open.) Pain intensifies when anxiety goes unchecked. Anxiety is reduced by establishing a warm, understanding relationship.

The Placebo Effect

The placebo effect is an integral part of the doctor-patient relationship. It often represents an extension of this relationship beyond the direct interpersonal exchange. Beecher showed the placebo to be effective in approximately 35% of cases.[12] Other studies have recorded 60% to 85% incidence of pain relief with placebos.[13] Dentists who understand the significance of the placebo on pain perception can make use of this principle. Should medication be indicated, it should be prescribed in a positive manner emphasizing that the patient will feel more relaxed and be better able to tolerate the dental procedure. The doctor need not prescribe a large dose of the drug and thereby risk an increase in side effects. Instead he or she should utilize the placebo effect to augment the pharmacologic influence of the agent. Trieger et al have shown that the significant effects of low-dose nitrous oxide–oxygen sedation in the conscious patient, which serve to produce "relative analgesia," are related largely to its placebo action.[14] True analgesia (absence of pain) for the patient receiving nitrous oxide requires unconsciousness.

The placebo reactor has been characterized further as a more extroverted personality who is more likely to have somatic symptoms when under stress and tends to use drugs more frequently. Psychologic tests show that people who respond more consistently to placebos have greater anxiety; however, most patients are not always consistent and at times react to a placebo while at other times they do not.[11]

Accessibility of professional attention also lessens anxiety. Frequently, dentists will be told by patients that their severe toothaches suddenly stopped when they made an appointment to be treated. Facial and head pain create a higher "quotient" of anxiety because of the patient's concern for the significance of such pain. Once the source of the pain is identified, the anxiety diminishes and the pain subsides.

Distraction: Audio Analgesia, Hypnosis

Distraction is commonly used to lessen pain. Audio analgesia, which provides a high-intensity sound stimulus, serves to distract the patient and minimize pain perception in a significant number of patients.[15] Hypnosis also serves to concentrate the patient's attention and thus interfere with the perception of pain. Hypnosis has been widely and effectively used presurgery and postsurgery, as well as for a larger number of nonsurgical complaints, with varying degrees of success. In practical experience, hypnosis for major surgery requires a patient with high motivation and concentration, with the capability of achieving a deep level of trance. Estimates are that only 5% of the population is able to achieve this goal.[16]

For minor surgery and general dental treatment successful use of hypnosis is considerably higher. Many dentists have utilized nitrous oxide–oxygen sedation techniques to serve the induction process for hypnosis. In this technique, the dentist can often reliably predict the sequence of sensory alternations and use this approach to reinforce rapport and establish a trance more readily. The effects of hypnosis have been only partially reversed by the narcotic antagonist naloxone hydrochloride.[17]

Acupuncture

Listening to a Chinese expert describe the workings of acupuncture reminds one of the early Greek exposition of the vital humors. It sounds remarkably similar to a Chinese interpretation of the phlogiston theory. Being almost in the twenty-first century and sophisticated in the ways of scientific endeavor and reason, we can readily recognize that these effects are induced by a belief in their effectiveness.

One cannot fault the Chinese or any other populace for seeking relief of physical and mental pain and suffering by whatever means available. Even in our modern society where so much is still unknown about the causes and courses of human diseases, we too do the best we can with our limited medications and therapies; beyond this point we offer only palliative or supportive care, including prayer and compassion.

Let us hypothesize that "acupuncture is a placebo." In patients as a group we have seen that placebos have a consistent therapeutic effect—statistically, 30% to 35%. This is also remarkably similar to results with hypnosis where approximately one third of patients make excellent subjects. Diseases such as asthma, peptic ulcers, spastic constipation, and hypertension, which respond well to hypnosis, are known to have a significant emotional component and are subject to considerable periodicity of remissions and exacerbations.

Consider further the "induction" process that did attend the use of acupuncture for anesthesia in China when it was first introduced to the West:

1. The patient must voluntarily elect this as the method of choice.
2. The patient is "conditioned" both by readings from Mao and by a week of "breathing exercises" (as in the case of the man who underwent removal of a lung segment) prior to surgery.
3. Upon entering the operating room the patient was met by a number of doctors, nurses, acupuncturists, and assistants, all expecting his favorable reaction.

4. The induction process became intensified as the needles were positioned and then either twirled manually or connected to a low-intensity source of direct current for a period of approximately 20 minutes.

Wall, who is the co-developer of the widely accepted "gate-control theory of pain," asserts that acupuncture's effectiveness as an anesthetic is due to hypnosis.[18] For Wall, the key factor suggesting this conclusion is that the procedure is not used on children in China, despite the fact that all major neural mechanisms are functioning by the age of 5. He says, "Children who are highly suggestible in some ways are not open to the sophisticated transfer of responsibility which is required for hypnosis. Children are not placebo reactors. In the West, they have not had time to learn our general belief that the syringe needle transmits relief of suffering. In China, it appears that children have not had time to learn that the acupuncture needle has the same magical properties." In attributing acupuncture's anesthetic effect to hypnosis he further concludes that it "in no way dismisses or diminishes the value of acupuncture."[18]

Man and Chen have proposed that the basis of acupuncture anesthesia is produced by the "gate-control" pain mechanism. As a result of the mild stimulation of peripheral nerves by the acupuncture needle, the large A-beta fibers are stimulated. "This produces a steady stream of nonpain impulses which closes the gate in the substantia gelatinosa, thus preventing pain impulses from passing through."[19] These researchers cite a problem with the gate-control theory as postulated by Melzack and Wall[20] in that the latter's theory was applicable to spinal nerves. The substantia gelatinosa of the dorsal horn of the spinal cord terminates in the medulla. Pain arising from the face and head would not be channeled to spinal nerves. Instead, Man and Chen propose that A-beta fibers send branches to the nuclei gracilis and cuneatus where they are relayed via the bulbothalamic tract to the ventral posterolateral nuclei of the thalamus. They thus postulate a "second gate" in the thalamus that can be closed to stop all pain impulses from any part of the body. Placing acupuncture needles in areas covered by the cranial nerves sends nonpain impulses directly to the thalamus without having to close the spinal cord gate in the substantia gelatinosa. Man and Chen claim that any one spot on the body surface can be used to produce "anesthesia" of all peripheral nerves. To emphasize their point they indicate that while acupuncture may eliminate pain it does not block other sensations. The Chinese claim an overall success of 90% with acupuncture, but knowledge of the exact mechanism of action is still problematic.[20]

Studies by Pomerantz, Cheng, and Law have shown that acupuncture causes the release of brain endorphins, which produce analgesia in animals and man.[21] This effect can be largely blocked by the narcotic antagonist naloxone hydrochloride. Thus a more reasonable explanation of the effect of acupuncture is available. It would appear that the exact location of the acupuncture meridians is less important than the irritation of the needles over a period of 15 to 20 minutes. This is generally done by manual manipulation or by low-voltage direct current attached to the needles.

In dentistry and oral surgery, Chao reported an overall success rate of 78% by using acupuncture.[22] His study began with the use of twelve classic acupuncture points and gradually eliminated all but two (Hoku) points. The analgesic effect remained constant.

Gate Control Theory of Pain

The gate control theory, first elucidated by Melzack and Wall,[20] suggests that inhibitory mechanisms exist in the central nervous system (CNS) that control pain. Older theories considered pain as a specific sensory experience mediated from pain receptors through nerve fibers going directly to the brain. This theory did not adequately explain certain common pathologic pain problems such as causalgia, phantom limb pain, and peripheral neuralgias. Evidence suggested that the amount and quality of perceived pain are determined by many psychologic variables in addition to sensory stimuli.

Anatomically, large myelinated fibers (A-beta), which are fast-conducting, carry nonpain impulses set off by mild stimuli. These fibers act to inhibit pain signals that travel via the smaller (C) fibers to the spinal cord. A specific area in the dorsal horn of the spinal cord is identified as the substantia gelatinosa. From this area afferent signals are relayed to the brain. The substantia gelatinosa has been recently recognized to be made up of at least six cell layers. Cell density, size, and shape vary in these several layers. It has been shown by Heavner[23] and by others that anesthesia induces changes in specific cells in these laminae. All general anesthetics caused depression of both spontaneous and evoked discharges of neurons in laminae IV, V, and VI. This depression was time- and dose-related and paralleled the clinical course of anesthesia. Analgesic agents such as morphine had little or no effect on these structures.

In recent years trigeminal neurons of the nucleus caudalis have been studied and shown to extend to cervical levels and to be continuous with the dorsal horn—the area of Melzack and Wall's "gate". Seventy-five percent nitrous oxide was found to suppress the spontaneous firing frequency of these trigeminal nociceptors and facilitate cutaneous receptor activity, thus showing a differential effect of nitrous oxide on the trigeminal neurons analogous to its effects on cells of the dorsal horn.[24]

Melzack and Wall write of a "central control trigger" wherein the brain activates descending efferent fibers that can influence afferent conduction.[20] Thus, the brain's activities subserving attention, emotion, and memories of past experiences exert control over the sensory input. This is the mechanism that explains the significance of the perceived pain and enables the organism to discern different properties of the stimulus and establish its precise location. Melzack and Wall dismiss the concept of any one "pain center" in the brain and propose that the thalamus, limbic system, hypothalamus, brainstem reticular formation, and parietal and frontal cortices are all implicated in pain perception. "The stimulation of a single tooth re-

sults in the eventual activation of no less than five distinct brainstem pathways".[20]

One important basis of pain control may be the anxiety-relieving effects of premedication acting on the brain, particularly in the areas of the limbic and reticular activating systems. This would serve to modify the efferent impulses to the "gate" and make local anesthesia much more effective. Repeatedly, patients are found with acute toothache that precludes comfortable treatment with local anesthetic block or infiltration alone; the addition of an intravenous sedative then allows successful pain-free manipulation.

Anxiety-reducing drugs involve the cyclic adenosine monophosphate phosphodiesterase (cyclic AMP) system in the brain. Benzodiazepine drugs such as diazepam (Valium) inhibit cyclic AMP activity. Serotonin antagonism, which also reduces anxiety, is produced by the benzodiazepines and barbiturates.[25,26]

Neurotransmitters in Pain Control[27]

All neurologic activity involves molecular changes. The hallmark of life itself is the excitability of cells. When these processes cease there is death. When these processes falter there is disease. When they function normally all cellular activities are coordinated and integrated into growth, development, creativity, and achievement.

Barchas et al write of "behavioral neurochemistry".[28] They offer a number of examples to show how neuroregulators act to adapt to environmental influences.

All the techniques we use to modify excitability, whether they be local or general anesthesia, hypnosis or behavior modification, placebo or compassion, require neurochemical change. Sigmund Freud, the father of psychiatry, always maintained that ultimately we would find a physical basis for neuroses and psychoses and indeed for all human thought and behavior.

A historical look at neurotransmission[29] (Table 2-1) shows that epinephrine was first isolated in 1898 by John Abel of Johns Hopkins University. J.N. Langley, using an extract from

Table 2-1. History of neurotransmission

YEAR	RESEARCHER	FINDING
1898	John Abel	Epinephrine isolated
1901	JN Langley	Sympathetic/parasympathetic and somatic nervous systems
1902	TR Elliot	"Neural communication by chemical transmitters"
1907	Dixon	Vagus liberates muscarine-like substance
1914	Sir Henry Dale	"Parasympathominetic" esterase
1921	Otto Loewi	Acetylcholine produced neural responses
1930	Walter Cannon	"Sympathin E and sympathin I"
1946	Von Euler	Norepinephrine as transmitter
1950	Kline	Reserpine blocks norepinephrine
1950	Lehman	Chlorpromazine (Thorazine) and the dopamine system
1960	Cotzias	Dopamine-levodopa for Parkinson's disease
1964	Li	Beta-lipotropin and beta-endorphin
1969	Reynolds	Opioid receptors
1974	Pert and Synder; Goldstein; Simon	Endorphins
1976	Udenfried	"Pro-opiocortin"
1977	Spector	"Morphine-like compound" (MLC)
1978	Ehrenpreis and Balgot	D-phenylalanine prolongs enkaphalin effect
1979	Goldstein	Dynorphin

the adrenal gland, stimulated various organs innervated by sympathetic nerves; on this basis he distinguished sympathetic, parasympathetic, and somatic nervous systems in 1901. It was recognized that autonomic systems consisted of postganglionic adrenergic sympathetic fibers.

In 1902, T.R. Elliot suggested that epinephrine was released from nerves when stimulated—he enunciated the concept of "neural communication by means of chemical transmitters." In 1907 Dixon suggested that the vagus nerve liberated a muscarine-like substance, and in 1914 Sir Henry Dale, after reinvestigating the properties of acetylcholine, introduced the term *parasympathomimetic*. He postulated that acetylcholine's extremely brief action was due to rapid destruction by an esterase in the tissues. He contrasted this with the relatively longer action of the neurotransmitter substance associated with the sympathetic system.

Otto Loewi in 1921 finally proved that chemical transmission in autonomic nerves by acetylcholine produced neural responses. Although acetylcholine had been known for over 50 years, its isolation and study had been ex-

tremely difficult because of its rapid hydrolysis by acetylcholinesterase, which is also present in high concentration wherever acetylcholine exists. Earlier studies indicated that anesthetics generally depress central cholinergic activity in mammals.[30] In 1978 a study had shown that different anesthetics, (e.g. halothane, enflurane, and ketamine), affect different specific brain areas and produce a change in the turnover rate of acetylcholine. More importantly, a causal relationship was demonstrated between the change in neurochemical transmitter acetylcholine at the specific brain site induced by the anesthetic and electrophysiologic effects as monitored from the brain.

During the 1930s Walter Cannon and others reported finding "sympathin," which was capable of increasing blood pressure and heart rate. They later described an excitatory substance "sympathin E," and an inhibitory substance, "sympathin I."

In 1946 Von Euler proposed norephinephrine as *the* chemical transmitter for the sympathetic system and indicated that sympathetic nerve stimulation may also liberate small quantities of epinephrine itself. For many years these three agents were believed to be the only neurotransmitters.

Then the substance dopamine, known to be involved in the formation of norepinephrine and epinephrine, was thought not only to be an intermediary but also to serve as a specific neurotransmitter in its own right. It was considered one of the greatest discoveries in the treatment of neurologic disease. In 1960 Cotzias treated patients with Parkinson's disease, who show a deficiency of dopamine in their basal ganglia, with levodopa. Levodopa produces dramatic results by controlling the tremor and cogwheel rigidity of Parkinson's patients. Prior to this, reserpine and chlorpromazine hydrochloride (Thorazine) were shown to tranquilize by influencing this dopamine transmitter system.

The pharmacologic management of serious psychiatric disease over the past 30 years has been predicated on the use of drugs that modify dopaminergic transmission. It is dramatic to see a schizophrenic patient who had discontinued daily chlorpromazine or haloperidol (Haldol) medication begin to redevelop frightening hallucinations after a week to ten days. This type of pharmacologic approach has greatly changed the need for long-term hospitalization of many psychotic patients. Other advances in psychiatric diseases await better understanding of neurotransmitter substances.

The benzodiazepines are a group of agents with wide therapeutic application as tranquilizers, anticonvulsants, hypnotics, and muscle relaxants. The main representative of this group of drugs is diazepam (Valium). Recently, specific benzodiazepine receptor sites have been identified in the CNS.[31] These sites are located primarily in the synaptic membrane fraction on the cell surface and not within the cell. The greatest concentration of these stereospecific receptors was found in the cerebral cortex, followed by the hypothalamus, and continued at decreasing concentrations caudally in the brain and spinal cord. A similar density distribution exists for receptors to the neurotransmitter gamma amino butyric acid (GABA), which supports the importance of this neurotransmitter in the action of benzodiazepines. The GABA receptor, however, does not appear to be the diazepam-specific binding site.

Tricyclic antidepressants, the major agents used in treating psychiatric depression today, form major groups. One group serves to control psychomotor agitation and has a high incidence of sedation—this group works by inhibiting serotonin uptake. The second group tends to overcome retarded depressive states by producing psychomotor activation—this group works by inhibiting the uptake of norepinephrine. Alpha noradrenergic receptor sites are readily identified in the brain. Sedative and hypnotic drugs act by blocking these receptor sites. The tricyclics show a close correlation between reducing psychomotor agitation and their affinity for alpha adrenergic binding sites in brain membranes.[32,33] Guilleman wrote of Reynolds finding a group of cells in the periventricular and periaqueductal gray areas of the brain, which when stimulated electrically produced profound analgesia equal to large doses of morphine.[34] This area was subsequently identified as the site of action by morphine. In very short order, Goldstein[35] at Stanford, Simon[36] at New York University, and Pert and Synder[37] of Johns Hopkins demonstrated these opiate receptors and theorized the presence of naturally occurring endogenous opiates to explain the presence of such highly specific receptors in mammals (see Table 2-1). Hughes et al in 1974 at the University of Aberdeen isolated opiate-like factors that they called enkephalins.[38] Terenius at the University of Uppsala independently identified morphine-like factors in brain extracts.[39] Other researchers searched for alternate functions. Kastin suggested that methionine or metenkephalin may facilitate learning. Frank, McCarthy, and Liebeskind showed that the seizure activity, or "wet-dog shakes," caused by injection of metenkephalin and leucine enkephalins, was distinct from areas of analgesic effects.[40]

A decade before the enkephalins were identified, Li from the University of California at San Francisco isolated the pituitary beta-lipotropin—a 91 amino acid polypeptide chain.[41] The amino acid sequence of the much smaller peptide, metenkephalin, matches a segment of the beta-lipotropin. Li imported a large number of camel pituitaries—the camel is known to be a pain-insensitive animal—and then extracted a 31 amino acid segment of lipotropin. The resulting compound was named beta endorphin and was found to be 48 times more potent than morphine when injected into the brain of experimental animals and three times more potent when injected intravenously. Simon at New York University is credited with coining the term *endorphin* for "morphine within."[36]

Other researchers isolated endorphins from other animals—mainly from the pituitary's pars intermedia. They identified alpha, beta, gamma, and delta endorphins, which showed varying effects: for example, alpha endorphins injected into rats produced 15 to 30 minutes of analgesia, chiefly of the head and neck region, reduced body temperature, and tranquilized the animal for 30 to 60 minutes. Beta endorphins produced profound analgesia for several hours, lowered body temperature and, depending on the dose, caused a catatonic state. Gamma endorphins did *not* produce analgesia but raised body temperature and made rats agitated and violent. Delta endorphins account for virtually all the opiate-like activity of the pituitary gland, which is almost devoid of enkephalin. ACTH and beta endorphin are probably derived from the same larger precursor molecule and both are released into the circulation at times of stress.[42]

Because of the wide variety of effects shown in the relationship of beta endorphins to behavior, an intense interest in psychiatric research has been generated. The intravenous injection of beta endorphin into a small number of psychotic patients in an uncontrolled study by Kline and Lehman (who developed reserpine and chlorpromazine, respectively, in the 1950s), yielded inconclusive results.[43] Laski of Einstein Medical College in New York was himself injected with beta endorphin and reported "a spaced-out, floating feeling" and a sensation of "perplexity." His mouth became dry, he became sleepy 4 hours after infusion, and his blood pressure fell to 80/40 for a number of hours. Watson et al, in a double-blind study, showed that naloxone reduced auditory hallucinations in schizophrenics.[44]

Endorphins may play a significant role in narcotic addition. It is theorized that exogenous opiates suppress endogenous opiate synthesis. Stopping the narcotic abruptly in the face of decreased endorphin leads to withdrawal symptoms.

Relief of intractable pain has been produced in human patients by stimulation of electrodes permanently implanted in the periventricular and periaqueductal gray areas. This relief was blocked by naloxone and also showed characteristic development of tolerance with repetitive stimulation.[45-48] Opiate receptors have been located in a number of areas, such as in the spinal cord (laminae I and II), in the substantia gelatinosa–spinal tract of the fifth cranial nerve, and in the nuclei of the solitary tract (commissuralis and ambiguous), which serve vagal responses, respiration, cough suppression, orthostatic hypotension, nausea and vomiting, and inhibition of gastric secretion, as well as in other areas controlling euphoria, miosis, etc.[49]

Udenfried of the Roche Institute of Molecular Biology had discovered that the original 91 peptide beta lipotropin described by Li is preceded by a much longer peptide molecule. This has been confirmed by others and is being called "pro-opiocortin" because it it is also a precursor to ACTH. This huge compound (which is 10 times that of beta endorphin) is released from the pituitary at times of stress. It divides into segments that affect a variety of neurohumoral mechanisms.

Spector at the Roche Institute of Molecular Biology discovered a nonpeptide morphine-like compound (MLC) in brain extracts, urine, and human cerebrospinal fluid.[50] This substance is 100 times more potent than morphine. It produced catatonic states when minute amounts were injected into rats. However, the reaction was not preventable or reversible with naloxone as it is with morphine or the endorphins.[51] Thus, morphine-like compound may constitute yet another neurotransmitter dealing with pain perception. Jacquet described two types of opiate receptors based on their response to the different dextro and levo forms of morphine.[52,53] The first type is highly stereospecific; these receptors are blocked by naloxone and mediate morphine analgesia. He suggested that their natural ligands are the endogenous endorphins. Receptors of the second type, possessing a low degree of stereospecificity and not being blocked by naloxone, mediate the syndrome of hyperexcitability and explosive motor behavior seen after direct microinjection of morphine into certain CNS sites. This latter effect is similar to abstinence syndrome and suggests a relationship in opiate dependence.

The current high interest in the neurophysiology of pain has led to yet another important recent discovery. A derivative of the naturally occurring nucleotide cyclic guanosine 3′, 5′ monophosphate (GMP), when administered directly into the CNS, produces a high level of analgesia without inducing sedation, depressing respiration, or altering either awareness or locomotor activity.[54] The analgesic properties are neither prevented nor reversed by naloxone. Cyclic GMP is ubiquitously present in all mammals with higher concentration found in the brain and certain organs. It has been linked to a role as a neurotransmitter in muscarinic cholinergic activity in the CNS and in the superior cervical ganglion. While it apparently plays a role in pain perception, cyclic GMP's mechanism of action is decidedly different from the opiates and remarkably free of their depressant effects.

Ehrenpreis at Chicago Medical School reported on the effect of administering the amino acid D-phenylalanine to mice. It apparently caused inhibition of carboxypeptidase A—an enzyme known to degrade enkephalin. These mice showed increased tolerance to pain and increased enkephalin levels.

It is most likely that the endorphins will be shown to be significant neurotransmitters for many neuroendocrine functions. The enkephalins are identified with mediation of pain. Is it possible that they provide for enhanced survival of the species by allowing most otherwise painful experience to be accommodated? Do they serve to dampen the pain after a while, much like other neural mechanisms show accommodation and increasing tolerance? Do they serve as a euphoriant or pleasure source or as a reward mechanism?

It has been noted that long-distance runners experience a kind of rapture after significant exertion of 3 to 4 miles or 15 to 20 minutes. They become euphoric and feel as if they could go on forever. They risk confronting traffic and other hazards with a sense of invincibility. Many runners speak of feeling "high" for a long period after the run is over. Indeed if this constitutes a back-up survival system taking over after the early adrenaline response is exhausted and lactic acid rises to painful levels, it could serve to blunt the pain and enable the animal to continue his or her flight or fight. Enkephalins have also been shown to inhibit the release of substance "P" from afferent neuron terminals and thereby to decrease nociception.[55]

We may some day soon come to understand how anesthesia really works. Recently it was demonstrated in mice that nitrous oxide at 55% significantly reduced the painful response to phenylquinone—a very irritating drug.[56] This effect was blocked by naloxone. This analgesic effect was attributed to nitrous oxide causing the release of endogenous endorphins. I have been unimpressed with our own limited attempts to demonstrate this relationship in humans. Using an electric pulp tester, threshold pain levels went unchanged despite 55% nitrous oxide for more than 45 minutes. Usually the subjective effects of nitrous oxide are noted within a minute after beginning inhalation. This is incompatible with the slower onset we recognize for endorphine release. Several recent reports substantiate that naloxone does not antagonize nitrous oxide anesthesia or other general anesthetics and therefore is not mediated by the endorphin-enkephalin system.[57,58]

Zuniga recently reported elevation of beta endorphin in specific brain nuclei in rats exposed to higher concentrations (60%-80%) of nitrous oxide.[59] Willer et al find that the analgesic effect of nitrous oxide is a nonspecific depressant action on the transmission of nociceptive messages, independent of pain-suppressive endogenous endorphins.[60]

Goodale proposes a unified hypothesis for oral pain, which identifies "substance P" as the common denominator, released from nerve terminals in the trigeminal nucleus, upon noxious stimulation.[61] Neurons then relay to higher brain centers for conscious proprioception and also to peripheral areas that evoke autonomic reactions to pain. Interference with substance P neurotransmission provides analgesia. Drugs such as narcotics, enkephalins, prostaglandins, and others are known to inhibit substance P. A third member of the opioid peptide clan has been identified and named *dynorphin*.[62,63]

Summary

The significance of pain in dentistry is responsible for the considerable incidence of neglect and suffering despite the availability of professional care. In legend, song, and cartoon the fear of dentistry permeates and reflects the meaning of pain in our culture. Such cultural influences are coupled with early learned experiences that accentuate the anxieties attending dental care. To offset these pervading influences, dentists use a number of psychologic and pharmacologic approaches to decrease anxiety and lessen pain perception. The placebo effect, properly used, is a valuable adjunct in patient management, as is distraction, audio analgesia, hypnosis, acupuncture, and electroanesthesia.

The "gate-control" theory of pain has done much to explain the many variables associated with pain perception. Neurohumoral and neurotransmitters such as the enkephalins, endorphins, "substance P," and others promise to provide better answers to questions of pain and anxiety control.

References

1. Wolff HG, Wolf SM: *Pain,* Springfield, Ill, 1958, Charles C Thomas.
2. Ayer WA, Hirschman RD: *Psychology and Dentistry,* Springfield, Ill, 1972, Charles C Thomas.
3. Melzack R, Scott TH: The effects of early experience on the response to pain, *J Comp Physiol* 50:155, 1957.
4. Jessner L, Blom FE, Waldfogel S: Emotional implications of tonsillectomy and adenoidectomy on children, *Psychoanal Study Child* 7:126, 1952.
5. Baldwin DC: An investigation of psychological and behavioral response to dental extractions in children, *J Dent Res* 45 (6):1637-1651, 1966.
6. Trieger N, Bernstein N: Good child, bad tooth, *Oral Surg Oral Med Oral Pathol* 16(3):261-270, 1963.
7. Beecher HK: Pain in men wounded in battle, *Ann Surg* 123:98-105, 1946.
8. Beecher HK: Relationship of significance of wound to pain experienced. *JAMA* 161(17): 1609-1613, 1956.
9. Beecher HK: *Measurements of subjective responses: quantitative effects of drugs,* New York, 1959, Oxford University Press.
10. Egbert LD et al: Reduction of post-operative pain by encouragement and instruction to patients: a study of doctor-patient rapport, *N Engl J Med* 270:825, 1964.
11. Egbert LD: Psychological support for surgical patients. In Abram, HS, editor: *Psychological aspects of surgery—International Psychiatry Clinics,* Boston, 1967, Little, Brown & Co.
12. Beecher HK: The powerful placebo, *JAMA* 159:1602, 1955.
13. Kolodny AK, McLoughlin PT: *Comprehensive approach to therapy of pain,* Springfield, Ill, 1966, Charles C Thomas.
14. Trieger N et al: Nitrous oxide—a study of physiological and psychomotor effects, *J Am Dent Assoc* 82(1):142-150, 1971.
15. Weisbroad RL: Audio analgesia revisited, *Anesth Prog* 16(1):8-14, 1969.
16. Freese AS: Hypnosis without ritual—a medical tool, *Med World News* Feb 2, 1973.
17. Frid M, Singer F: Hypnotic analgesia in conditions of stress is partially reversed by naloxone, *Psychopharmacology* 63:211-215, 1979.
18. Wall PD: Hypnosis held anesthetic base of acupuncture, *Hosp Trib* Feb 26, 1973.
19. Man PL, Chen CH: Acupuncture "anesthesia": a new theory and clinical study, *Curr Ther Res* 14(7):390-394, 1972.
20. Melzack R, Wall PD: Pain mechanism: a new theory, *Science* 150:971, 1965.
21. Pomeranz B, Cheng R, Law P: Acupuncture reduces electrophysiological and behaviorial responses to noxious stimuli: pituitary is implicated, *Exp Neurol* 54:172, 1977.

22. Chao MCF: Acupuncture in dentistry and oral surgery. TriService General Hospital, Taipei, Taiwan. (Personal communication, 1976.)

23. Heavner JE: The spinal cord dorsal horn, *Anesthesiology* 38 (1):1-3, 1973.

24. Kitahata LM, McAllister RF, Taub A: Identification of central trigeminal nociceptors and the effects of nitrous oxide. *Anesthesiology* 38(1): 12-19, 1973.

25. Beer B. et al: Cyclic adenosine monophosphate phosphodiestrase in brain: effect on anxiety, *Science* 176:428-430, 1972.

26. Wise CD, Berger BD, Stein L: Benzodiazepines: anxiety-reducing activity by reduction of serotonin turnover in the brain, *Science* 177:180-183, 1972.

27. Trieger N: New neurotransmitters in pain control, *Anesth Prog* 26(3):66-71, 1979.

28. Barchas JD et al: Behavioral neurochemistry: neuroregulators and behavioral states, *Science* 200:964-973, 1978.

29. Mayer SE: *Neurohumoral transmission and the autonomic nervous system.* In Gilman et al, editors: *The Pharmacologic Basis of therapeutics,* New York, 1988, Macmillan.

30. Hanin I: Anesthetics and central cholenergic function—a perspective, *Anesthesiology* 48(1): 1-3, 1978 (editorial).

31. Mohler H, Okada T: Benzodiazepines receptor: demonstration in the central nervous system, *Science* 198:849, 1977.

32. U'Prichard D et al: Tricyclic antidepressants: therapeutic properties and affinity for alpha noradrenergic receptor binding sites in the brain, *Science* 199:197, 1978.

33. de Montigny C, Aghajanian GK: Tricyclic antidepressants: long-term treatment increased responsivity of rat forebrain post synaptic neurons to serotonin, *Science* 202:1303-1305, 1978.

34. Guillemin R: Peptides in the brain: the new endocrinology of the neuron, *Science* 202: 390-402, 1978.

35. Goldstein A: Opioid peptides (endorphins) in pituitary and brain, *Science* 193:1081-1086, 1976.

36. Simon EJ: The intriguing endorphins, Medical Newsmagazine 22(1):47-49, 1978.

37. Pert CB, Pasternak GW, Synder SH: Opiate agonists and antagonists discriminated by receptor binding in brain, *Science* 182:1359-1361, 1975.

38. Hughes J et al: Identification of two related pentapeptides from the brain with potent opiate agonist activity, *Nature* 258:577-579, 1975.

39. Terenius L: *Characteristics and function of opioids,* Amsterdam, 1978, Elsevier.

40. Frank H, McCarthy BC, Liebeskind JC: Different brain areas mediate analgesic and epileptic properties of enkephalin, *Science* 200:335-336, 1978.

41. Li CH, Chung D: Isolation and structure of an untriakontapeptide with opiate activity from camel pituitary glands, *Nature* 208:1093, 1965.

42. Synder SH: Opiate receptors in the brain in physiology in medicine, *N Engl J Med* 296(5): 266-271, 1977.

43. Kline NS: Clinical experience with iproniazid (Marsilid), *J Clin Exp Psychopathol* 19(suppl): 72-78, 1958.

44. Watson SJ et al: Effects of naloxone on schizophrenia: reduction in hallucinations in a subpopulation of subjects, *Science* 201:73-75, 1978.

45. Hosobuchi Y, Adams JE, Linchitz R: Pain relief by electrical stimulation of the central gray matter in humans and its reversal by naloxone, *Science* 197:183-186, 1977.

46. Akil H, Mayer DJ, Liebeskind JC: Antagonism of stimulation—produced analgesia by naloxone, a narcotic antagonist, *Science* 191:961-962, 1976.

47. Akil H et al: Enkephalin-like material elevated in ventricular cerebrospinal fluid in pain patients after analgetic focal stimulation, *Science* 201:463-465, 1978.

48. Hosobuchi Y et al: Stimulation of human periaqueductal gray matter for pain relief increases immunoreactive B-endorphin in ventricular fluid, *Science* 203:279-281, 1979.

49. Neale JN et al: Enkephalin-containing neurons visualized in spinal cord cell cultures, *Science* 201:467-469, 1978.

50. Spector S, Parker CW: Morphine-like compound in brain extracts, *Science* 168:1347, 1970.

51. Gintzler AR, Gershon MD, Spector S: A nonpeptide morphine-like compound: immunocytochemical localization in the mouse brain, *Science* 199:447-448, 1978.

52. Jacquet YF, Marks N: The C-fragment of beta-lipotropin: an endogenous neuroleptic or antipsychotogen? *Science* 194:632-634, 1976.

53. Jacquet YF: Opiate effects after adrenocorticotropin or beta-endorphin injection in the pe-

riaqueductal gray matter of rats, *Science* 201: 1032-1034, 1978.

54. Cohn ML, Cohn M, Taylor FH: Guanosine 3', 5' monophosphate: a central nervous system regulator of analgesia, *Science* 199:319-322, 1978.

55. Frederickson RCA et al: Dual actions of substance P on nociception: possible role of endogenous opioids. Science 199:1359-1361, 1978.

56. Berkowitz BA, Ngai SH, Finch AD: Nitrous oxide "analgesia": resemblance to opiate action, *Science* 194:967-968, 1976.

57. Smith RA, Wilson M, Miller KW: Naloxone has no effect on nitrous oxide anesthesia, *Anesthesiology* 49:6-8, 1978.

58. Harper MH et al: Naloxone does not antagonize general anesthesia in the rat, *Anesthesiology* 39:311, 1978.

59. Zuniga JR: Evidence of central B-endorphin release and recovery after exposure to nitrous oxide, *Am Assoc Oral Maxillofac Surg,* 1985 (abstract).

60. Willer JC et al: Failure of naloxone to reverse nitrous oxide-induced depression of a brain stem reflex: an electrophysiologic and double-blind study in humans, *Anesthesiology* 63(5): 467-472, 1985.

61. Goodale DP: Inhibition of substance P release is the key to successful management of oral pain, *Anesth Prog* 29(4):103-107, 1982.

62. Bonica JJ, editor: *The management of pain,* ed 2, Philadelphia, 1990, Lea & Febiger.

63. Goldstein A et al: Dynorphin (1-13), an extraordinarily potent opioid peptide, *Proc Natl Acad Sci USA* 76:6666, 1979.

3

Pretreatment Patient Evaluation

The key to successful pain control management is patient evaluation, and the basis of this evaluation is the medical history. Fortunately, most patients who present to the dentist for treatment are healthy and can easily tolerate the anticipated stress. It is estimated that approximately 85% of patients treated in a general dental practice are in this category. However, this incidence changes dramatically in a referral practice and in a hospital-affiliated dental clinic where the patient's medical chart is usually available to assist in the evaluation before dental treatment.

No laboratory tests can substitute for a well-taken medical history. Most offices today make use of the patient questionnaire recommended by the American Dental Association (Fig. 3-1). These basic questions provide a good starting point for the assessment of each individual. Familiarity with concepts of cardiovascular and pulmonary physiology and pathology will prompt the dentist to ask further clarifying questions and seek a consultation with the patient's physician when indicated.

There are myriad diseases that may affect the way in which patients respond to stress, medication, and manipulative procedures. It is often better to analyze the problem and think in terms of the significance of the impairment due to the diseased organ system rather than to memorize a listing of specific conditions. The basic substrate upon which we must rely for safe and effective patient management and pain control in dentistry is the integrity of the cardiovascular system. Other disorders must be assessed as to

their influence or effect on this vital foundation (Fig. 3-2).

The cardiac output is primarily regulated by the oxygen demands of the tissues of the body. The immediate tissue response to hypoxia is vasodilation, and the delayed response is increased vascularity in the deprived tissues.[1]

Cardiovascular Disease

Anything that diminishes the functions of the heart compromises the safety and survival of the patient and affects management directly. Some cardiovascular problems are subsequently described.

VALVULAR HEART DISEASE

Defects of the valves between the chambers of the heart, by impeding flow (stenosis) or by allowing regurgitation, diminish the efficiency of the heart; in this way, congenital heart disease and rheumatic heart damage pose a threat to the long-range survival of the patient. Defective heart valves also pose a secondary problem because the greater likelihood of the localization of bacteria from the bloodstream on these damaged valves threatens an endocarditis.

In 1989 the *Medical Letter* updated The American Heart Association's recommendations for the prevention of bacterial (infective) endocarditis associated with dental treatment. ''Regimen A: Oral'' is indicated for most congenital heart diseases, rheumatic heart disease, or other acquired valvular heart disease. The regimen now involves oral amoxicillin 3 g 60 minutes before the procedure, followed by 1.5 g

Medical History Form

Date _____

Name _____
    Last   First   Middle

Home Phone (____) _____

Address _____
    Number, Street

Business Phone (____) _____

City _____ State _____ Zip Code _____

Occupation _____ Social Security No. _____

Date of Birth ___/___/___ Sex M F Height _____ Weight _____ Single _____ Married _____
    mo. day yr.

Name of Spouse _____ Closest Relative _____ Phone (____) _____

If you are completing this form for another person, what is your relationship to that person? _____

Referred by _____

For the following questions, *circle yes or no*, whichever applies. Your answers are for our records only and will be considered confidential. Please note that during your initial visit you will be asked some questions about your responses to this questionnaire and there may be additional questions concerning your health.

1. Are you in good health? . . . . Yes   No
2. Has there been any change in your general health within the past year? . . . . Yes   No
3. My last physical examination was on _____
4. Are you now under the care of a physician? . . . . Yes   No
   If so, what is the condition being treated? _____
5. The name and address of my physician(s) is _____
   _____
   _____
6. Have you had any serious illness, operation, or been hospitalized in the past 5 years? . . . . Yes   No
   If so, what was the illness or problem? _____
7. Are you taking any medicine(s) including non-prescription medicine?. . . . . Yes   No
   If so, what medicine(s) are you taking? _____
8. Do you have or have you had any of the following diseases or problems?
   a. Damaged heart valves or artificial heart valves, including heart murmur or rheumatic heart disease . . . . . . Yes   No
   b. Cardiovascular disease (heart trouble, heart attack, angina, coronary insufficiency, coronary occlusion, high blood pressure, arteriosclerosis, stroke) . . . . Yes   No
      1. Do you have chest pain upon exertion? . . . . Yes   No
      2. Are you ever short of breath after mild exercise or when lying down?. . . . . Yes   No
      3. Do your ankles swell? . . . . Yes   No
      4. Do you have inborn heart defects?. . . . . Yes   No
      5. Do you have a cardiac pacemaker? . . . . Yes   No
   c. Allergy . . . . Yes   No
   d. Sinus trouble . . . . Yes   No
   e. Asthma or hay fever . . . . Yes   No
   f. Fainting spells or seizures . . . . Yes   No
   g. Persistent diarrhea or recent weight loss . . . . Yes   No
   h. Diabetes . . . . Yes   No
   i. Hepatitis, jaundice or liver disease . . . . Yes   No
   j. AIDS or HIV infection . . . . Yes   No
   k. Thyroid problems . . . . Yes   No
   l. Respiratory problems, emphysema, bronchitis, etc. . . . . Yes   No
   m. Arthritis or painful swollen joints . . . . Yes   No
   n. Stomach ulcer or hyperacidity . . . . Yes   No
   o. Kidney trouble . . . . Yes   No
   p. Tuberculosis . . . . Yes   No
   q. Persistent cough or cough that produces blood . . . . Yes   No
   r. Persistent swollen glands in neck . . . . Yes   No
   s. Low blood pressure . . . . Yes   No
   t. Sexually transmitted disease . . . . Yes   No
   u. Epilepsy or other neurological disease . . . . Yes   No
   v. Problems with mental health . . . . Yes   No
   w. Cancer . . . . Yes   No
   x. Problems of the immune system . . . . Yes   No

Fig. 3-1. Health questionnaire recommended by the American Dental Association.   *Continued.*

9.	Have you had abnormal bleeding?.	Yes	No
	a. Have you ever required a blood transfusion?	Yes	No
10.	Do you have any blood disorder such as anemia?	Yes	No
11.	Have you ever had any treatment for a tumor or growth?	Yes	No
12.	Are you allergic or have you had a reaction to:		
	a. Local anesthetics	Yes	No
	b. Penicillin or other antibiotics	Yes	No
	c. Sulfa drugs	Yes	No
	d. Barbiturates, sedatives, or sleeping pills	Yes	No
	e. Aspirin	Yes	No
	f. Iodine	Yes	No
	g. Codeine or other narcotics	Yes	No
	h. Other _____		
13.	Have you had any serious trouble associated with any previous dental treatment?	Yes	No
	If so, explain _____		
	_____		
14.	Do you have any disease, condition, or problem not listed above that you think I should know about?	Yes	No
	If so, explain _____		
	_____		
15.	Are you wearing contact lenses?	Yes	No
16.	Are you wearing removable dental appliances?	Yes	No

Women

17.	Are you pregnant?	Yes	No
18.	Do you have any problems associated with your menstrual period?	Yes	No
19.	Are you nursing?	Yes	No
20.	Are you taking birth control pills?	Yes	No

Chief Dental Complaint _____

_____

I certify that I have read and understand the above. I acknowledge that my questions, if any, about the inquiries set forth above have been answered to my satisfaction. I will not hold my dentist, or any other member of his/her staff, responsible for any errors or omissions that I may have made in the completion of this form.

_____
Signature of Patient

For completion by the dentist.
Comments on patient interview concerning medical history: _____
_____
_____
_____

Significant findings from questionnaire or oral interview: _____
_____
_____
_____

Dental management considerations: _____
_____
_____
_____

_____   _____
(Date)   Signature of Dentist

Medical history update:

Date	Comments	Signature
_____	_____	_____
_____	_____	_____
_____	_____	_____
_____	_____	_____
_____	_____	_____

Fig. 3-1, cont'd. Health questionnaire recommended by the American Dental Association.

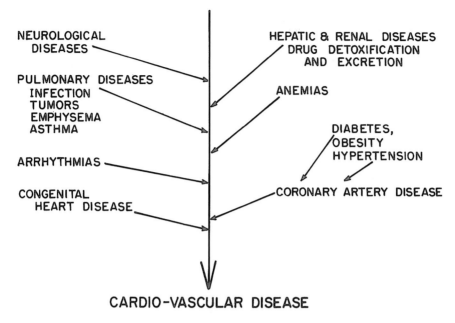

Fig. 3-2. Pretreatment patient evaluation considers those medical diseases or disorders that influence the basic integrity of the cardiovascular and pulmonary systems.

6 hours later. For patients allergic to amoxicillin or penicillin, erythromycin 1 g 2 hours before the procedure, followed by 500 mg 6 hours later, is advised.

Parenteral administration is recommended for patients with prosthetic heart valves—"Regimen B": ampicillin 2 g IM or IV 30 minutes before the procedure plus gentamicin 70 to 80 mg (based on 1.5 mg/kg IM or IV before the procedure). For patients allergic to penicillin: vancomycin 1 g IV, administered slowly over 60 minutes before the procedure. No further postoperative dosing is advised.[2]

Sadowsky and Kunzel,[3] in their study of dentist and physician compliance with the recommendations of the American Heart Association, reported considerable confusion and uncertainty about the use of subacute bacterial endocarditis (SBE) prophylaxis.

Since 1984, when recommendations were revised, after discussion with infectious disease consultants, the most critical period for prophylaxis was noted to be during the time when the bacteria were induced by the dental procedure. The consultants suggested that multiple postprocedure antibiotic doses were unwarranted. A compromise was reached by recommending that only one postoperative dose be given 6 hours later (in addition to the immediate preoperative administration). Thus, the latest recommendations provide for preoperative "loading" and one dose of antibiotics postoperatively. However, in an effort to broaden the spectrum of antibiotic effectiveness for patients at risk, ampicillin and, more recently, amoxicillin rather than penicillin has been designated as the agent of first choice.

Although much discussion and concern have focused on the prevention of infective endocarditis, very little teaching has been directed toward the recognition of signs and symptoms of SBE. Knowledge of the basic histopathology of heart valve damage did not seem to be translated into meaningful clinical information by the student or practitioner. The following vignette is offered to provide some discrete details about this disease and to respond more appropriately with a higher index of suspicion.

MD: Dr. Foster? This is Dr. Michaels calling. I'm a senior resident on the medical service at the General Hospital. We've just admitted a patient you treated in your dental office about 6 weeks ago. Do you recall a Mr. Cavanaugh?

DDS: Sure I do. He was the gentleman with a heart valve lesion that I premedicated with penicillin before I did a prophy and one extraction. I saw him again 1 week later and he was doing all right except for feeling a bit "washed out."

MD: Well, we admitted him to the hospital with a provisional diagnosis of subacute bacterial endocarditis. He has had a low-grade fever, up to 101° F, and several episodes of night sweats over the past few weeks. His blood cultures, drawn on admission to the hospital, are positive and growing a streptococcus that has not yet been completely identified.

DDS: I'm sorry to hear that, but I followed the recommendations of the American Heart Association. He got 2 g of oral penicillin 1 hour before my appointment and one 500-mg tablet every 6 hours for eight doses afterward.

MD: His infection may be from an organism that is not penicillin sensitive. Maybe due to an enterococcus like *Strep faecalis*, which is usually found in the GI tract and occasionally in the mouth also.

DDS: Should I have used another antibiotic?

MD: Hard to say—you followed the approved recommendations (prior to 1989). Of course, if he had a valve prosthesis, additional coverage would have been indicated. What would probably have been more important was to be more suspicious on your follow-up visit, especially since you noted that he was feeling "washed out," to use your own phrase.

DDS: What would I look for?

MD: Well, most of the early symptoms of SBE are subtle and gradual in onset and may not be very dramatic. The patient often reports malaise and a low-grade fever. The longer the infection goes on, the greater the damage to the heart and potentially to other organs.

DDS: Well, I'm not prepared to listen for cardiac murmurs—but is there anything else I can elicit on history or cursory examination?

MD: Petechiae are found in about 40% of patients, showing up on the conjunctiva, the palate, buccal mucosae, and skin of the extremities. Splinter hemorrhages—dark red, linear streaks—are seen under the nails. Because friable vegetations form on the infected heart valve leaflets, they may break off and become emboli, where they may end up causing infarction of that particular organ. For example, the pa-

tient may complain of a sudden onset of left upper abdominal pain if the spleen is infarcted. Emboli to the retina may cause sudden blindness; emboli to the coronaries may cause myocardial infarction. Strangely, a sudden personality change or other sudden neurologic deficit may be caused by emboli to the brain. Medical laboratory tests would be required to show the high incidence of kidney involvement with SBE (50%); most patients with chronic infection become anemic and have elevated erythrocyte sedimentation rate. There are other more specific lab tests, of course. *The single most important finding in infective endocarditis patients is the positive blood culture, which is found in over 90% unless the patient has received inadequate antibiotic treatment and the organism is only partially suppressed.*

DDS: What sort of treatment will Mr. Cavanaugh require?

MD: Once the organism is definitely identified and the proper antibiotic selected, he will require a prolonged course of intravenous antibiotics which may vary from 2 to 6 weeks depending upon his response to the treatment.

DDS: Thank you very much for the 'clinic,' Dr. Michaels. I hope Mr. Cavanaugh gets better soon. I'll be more on the alert in the future for patients I have to premedicate.

MD: Okay, I'll call and give you a follow-up next week. Goodbye.

CORONARY ARTERY DISEASE

Oxygenation and nutrition of the heart muscle fibers are dependent upon the coronary arteries' integrity and patency. Arteriosclerotic plaques cause narrowing of the lumen, which leads to ischemia of the myocardium and "angina pectoris." Nitroglycerin, taken for the symptomatic relief of anginal pains, produces peripheral vasodilation with pooling of blood in peripheral veins and thus temporarily reduces the work of the heart and the myocardial oxygen requirement.[4] The complete occlusion of a coronary vessel produces an infarction with subsequent loss of normal muscle function from scarring. Following myocardial infarction the cardiac output is reduced, as is the heart's capacity to respond to increased demands, and elective dental treatment should be deferred for at least 6 months. It has been shown that general anesthesia and the stress of major surgery lead to a significantly greater mortality rate during this period.[5] Emergency dental care may be required to relieve pain and acute infection, but this is best carried out under sedation and local anesthesia after appropriate consultation with the patient's physician.

Generally, two types of angina pectoris are recognized: one, referred to as *variant angina* or *Prinzmetal's angina,* is due to coronary artery spasm. It may exist independently or coexist with the atheromatous (obstructive) type. Adrenergic blocking drugs, such as propranolol hydrochloride (Inderal), serve the more common type of angina, which is caused by arteriosclerotic narrowing of the coronary arteries. In some patients Inderal may decrease the myocardial oxygen requirement. This is accomplished by reducing heart rate and lowering arterial pressure and cardiac output.[4] In patients with advanced heart disease, beta-blockade with propranolol is ill-advised and may precipitate congestive heart failure.

Another group of drugs used for the treatment of angina pectoris is the calcium channel blocking agents. These drugs, verapamil hydrochloride (Isoptin) and nifedipine (Procardia) work by interfering with the flow of calcium required in the excitation-contraction coupling of cardiac and smooth muscle. Calcium channel blockers thus dilate coronary and peripheral vessels and decrease cardiac contractility in addition to lowering blood pressure.[6] These agents are less effective in angina that is caused by fixed stenosis of coronary arteries, where the efficacy of angioplasty and coronary artery bypass surgery have been extensively employed.

DIABETES

There are a number of diseases that cause early and more rapid narrowing of the coronary vessels. Two of the commonest are diabetes mellitus and hypertension. Originally, diabetes was believed to be a metabolic disorder primarily affecting glucose metabolism. Now it is apparent that more serious underlying sequelae of diabetes are caused by pernicious action to the walls of blood vessels, which results in arteriosclerosis and impedance to normal flow and function. Insulin-dependent diabetes (type I, juvenile-onset, ketosis-prone, or labile diabetes) is pathogenically a distinct disorder from the non-insulin-dependent diabetes (type II, maturity-onset, or stable diabetes.)[7] Insulin-dependent diabetes is believed to be caused by autoimmune destruction of the insulin-producing (beta cells) of the pancreas, perhaps initiated by a viral infection.

The effect of the diabetic control and its influence on producing microangiopathy has been the subject of prolonged debate. Raskin et al showed significant reduction in capillary basement membrane thickness in well-controlled diabetics given insulin by continuous subcutaneous infusion when compared to a control group receiving conventional treatment— usually two injections of insulin daily.[8] Control was monitored by glycosylated hemoglobin levels that reflect long-term glucose levels rather than static samples.[9]

Diabetics have a significantly higher incidence of cardiovascular disease at a younger age than the normal population. Juvenile diabetics frequently have erratic blood sugar levels and are prone to develop hyperglycemic acidosis and dehydration, particularly in the presence of fever and infection. Their response to insulin may also vary widely and rapidly with the development of hypoglycemic shock and unconsciousness. The dental problems of such "brittle" diabetic children are often best managed in a hospital setting. Generally, the diabetic patient requiring an anesthetic is admitted to the hospital on the day before the operation in order to regulate the disease. On the morning of surgery the patient's insulin dosage is reduced to avoid the possibility of developing hypoglycemia while under anesthesia. Following recovery from anesthesia, the patient's blood sugar levels are elevated and rapidly acting insulin is given as required. Older patients with "maturity-onset diabetes" are frequently controlled by diet alone, or in combination with one of the oral hypoglycemic agents. These patients should be considered at greater risk because of their underlying degenerative cardiovascular disease. In addition, failure to eat normally before a dental appointment may result in lowering of the blood sugar level with attendant subtle changes such as irritability, mental confusion, and somnolence. The use of adjunctive sedative drugs may produce further depressive effects and should be used with caution.

HYPERTENSION

Hypertension also accelerates the development of artery-clogging deposits and increases the risk of heart attacks and cerebral vascular accidents (strokes). In only a small percentage of patients with hypertension is persistent elevation of systolic blood pressure (over 150 mm Hg) due to known causes such as advanced kidney disease. Rarely are aldosteronism (caused by a hormone that promotes retention of salt and water by the kidneys) and pheochromocytoma (a tumor of the adrenal glands that produces large quantities of norepinephrine and epinephrine) implicated.

In the great majority of patients with hypertension the cause is unknown (*essential hypertension*). It is currently believed that this latter form of hypertension is caused by abnormal activity of the CNS, which produces increased sympathetic blood vessel tone. The hypertensive patient's responses frequently resemble those normally brought about by exertion; heart rate and output rise with widespread constriction of the peripheral vessels and a resultant increase in blood pressure. Similar recurring or persistent changes are alleged to lead to a "resetting" of the carotid sinus and aortic arch pressure regulators (baroreceptors) with resultant hypertension. There is usually a strong familial history of hypertension in affected individuals.

It has been shown that the development of congestive heart failure in the hypertensive patient is six times more common than in the normotensive.[10] Whereas hypertension was formerly diagnosed primarily on the basis of an elevated diastolic pressure (above 95 mm Hg), Kannel et al showed that persistently elevated systolic pressure alone could be accurately predictive of a developing cardiac hypertrophy and, later, of congestive heart failure.[10] Conges-

tive failure is a lethal phenomenon with only 50% survival for 5 years. Early and sustained control of hypertension has been effective in preventing congestive heart failure.[10] Recent experiments with hypertensive rats suggest that the defect may lie in the smooth muscle of the blood vessel walls. These animals were selectively bred and described as genetically hypertensive. They were further stressed by exposure to intermittent neurogenic stimulation, and hypertension became apparent in 4 to 6 weeks. The aortas were studied and compared with those of a control group of animals: they showed a significant difference in the metabolism of cyclic AMP (adenosine 3', 5'-monophosphate phosphodiesterase). The hypertensive animals showed considerably less cyclic AMP, indicating much higher enzyme activity (phosphodiesterase) and breakdown of the cyclic AMP.[11] Cyclic AMP concentrations are inversely correlated with vascular smooth muscle tone.

It has been proposed that a natriuretic hormone in the body of genetically predisposed patients increases sodium ion excretion by blocking its reuptake by the kidney. At the same time, this hormone is believed to cause an increase in salt levels in other cells of the body in the presence of increased dietary salt intake. An ion transport system within the cell exchanges sodium for calcium ions—moving calcium out of the cell normally. If the intracellular sodium is elevated because of pump inhibition calcium may fail to move out and may serve to trigger muscle contraction.[12] This leads to greater contraction of smooth muscles in the arterioles and eventual structural changes making them more rigid. The arterioles are also shown to be more responsive to norepinephrine, resulting in sustained contraction.

In a large national study of nutrients and hypertension, McCarron et al reported that low calcium intake was the most consistent factor in hypertensive individuals.[13] Higher intakes of calcium, potassium, and sodium were associated with lower risk of hypertension. The authors conclude that hypertension may be a disease of nutritional deficiencies and not salt excess. They also hasten to add that these findings do not prove causality; they indicate potentially important relations between nutrients and blood pressure regulation in humans.

Hypertension is treated in a variety of ways: weight reduction and restriction of sodium intake are primary. A decrease in body fat lessens the burden on the heart. Drug therapy for hypertension is graduated: mild sedatives and tranquilizers are frequently prescribed for mild hypertension; thiazide diuretics, (chlorothiazide [Diuril], hydrochlorothiazide [Hydrodiuril], furosemide [Lasix], which increase the secretion of sodium by the kidneys, are also given to assist reduction of fluid and blood pressure elevation. More aggressive drug therapy is aimed at decreasing the activity of the sympathetic nervous system by interfering or blocking the action of norepinephrine. Reserpine, methyldopa (Aldomet), monamine oxidase inhibitors, and guanethidine (Ismeline) may be used to control severe hypertension.

Propranolal (Inderal) blocks beta-adrenergic receptors and produces reductions in systolic and diastolic pressures. Its sudden withdrawal in patients with atherosclerotic heart disease has been associated with an increased incidence of myocardial infarction. Other significant side effects include bradycardia, reduced exercise tolerance, congestive heart failure, and increased bronchial airway resistance. It may also block the sympathetic response to hypoglycemia.

A new group of antihypertensive agents known as "angiotensin-converting enzyme inhibitors" (e.g., enalapril maleate, Vasotec) recently became available. These drugs interfere with the conversion of angiotensin I to angiotensin II and suppress the renin-angiotensin-aldosterone system. These ACE agents have shown few significant side effects and have gained wide usage.

Special care in dental patient management for the hypertensive patient is indicated. Patients on the ganglionic antihypertensive blocking agents, (e.g., guanethidine), are prone to developing hypotension with rapid changes in position, so positional changes in the dental chair should be gradual; some time should be allowed for adaptation before the patient is sat upright and discharged. In general, hypertensive patients benefit from mild sedation during dental appointments. With the patient who is taking monoamine oxidase inhibitors, paradoxical hypertensive crisis or severe hypotensive episodes may occur with the administration of other sedative drugs such as narcotics or epinephrine.

DYSRHYTHMIAS—EFFECT ON HEART FUNCTION

While the normal heart beat is usually regular and approximately 70 to 80 per minute, considerable normal variation is seen in both rate and rhythm. Normal healthy young adults, monitored continuously, will show wide fluctuation in both rate and rhythm depending upon their activity, psychic stress, etc. One of the most common variations seen is tachycardia—a rate greater than 120 beats per minute. If the tachycardia is sustained for a long period of time the heart becomes taxed. At higher rates the ventricles have insufficient time to adequately fill with blood and cardiac output decreases. Irregularities of rhythm too are found in various disease states where the normal conduction system that triggers synchronous contractions of the atria and ventricles is disturbed. A presumptive diagnosis of several different dsyrhythmias is possible by palpation of the radial or carotid pulses. Whereas tachycardia, bradycardia (less than 60 beats per minute), and atrial fibrillation (an irregular beat) are readily discernible, other abnormalities require an electrocardiograph to confirm the diagnosis.

Chronic atrial fibrillation develops, with increasing age, in myocardial infarction and with congestive failure when the conduction system is disturbed; in association with rheumatic heart disease; and with hyperthyroidism. Atrial fibrillation should alert the clinician to the presence of significant underlying heart disease. It was found to be associated with a doubling of the overall mortality rate from cardiovascular disease.[14]

Such dysrhythmias must be viewed as evidence of a diseased heart, subject to the likelihood of further rapid changes, particularly in the face of great physical or emotional stress, hypoxia, and certain drugs. Ventricular fibrillation or cardiac arrests constitute an acute emergency requiring immediate recognition and resuscitation.

ANEMIA

To carry oxygen from the lungs to nourish the demands of all living body tissues is primarily the function of the red blood cell. The most common form of anemia is due to iron deficiency—usually caused by blood loss and inadequate replacement of iron stores in the body. Other causes are defective synthesis of new erythrocytes (hypoplastic bone marrow and maturation arrest) or the too-rapid breakdown of red blood cells (hemolysis). Inherited anemias include sickle cell disease (hemoglobin S) and hereditary spherocytosis, both of which produce abnormally shaped erythrocytes that are more vulnerable to mechanical fragility and are more rapidly destroyed in the body.

Deficiency of an enzyme (glucose-6-phosphate dehydrogenase [G6PD]) affects a large number of patients, particularly blacks and those of Mediterranean descent. When challenged by certain oxidant drugs (e.g., primaquine, para-aminosalicylic acid, phenacetin), these patients show hemolysis and more rapid destruction of erythrocytes. Thalassemia (Cooley's anemia) is also an inherited disease found primarily in peoples of the Mediterranean basin. All inherited forms of anemia also exist in lesser clinical forms designated as "traits." Regardless of the form of anemia, the net effect on the heart is a significantly greater burden to supply oxygenated blood to all vital tissues.

The normal level of hemoglobin is usually 12 to 16 g/100 ml (deciliter) of blood. Anesthesiologists arbitrarily insist upon a minimum of 10 g of hemoglobin preoperatively for any elective surgery and anesthesia. The heart of an anemic patient given depressant anesthetics is further compromised and function decreases to precarious levels.

Examples of Pretreatment Patient Evaluation

Patients with atherosclerotic heart disease who have survived a myocardial infarction and are not decompensated, are neither dyspneic on exertion nor orthopneic, have no evidence of peripheral edema such as ankle swelling, and whose chest pain is very infrequent and controllable by rest or nitroglycerin are usually best treated by intravenous premedication and a local anesthetic.

Nunn and Freeman[15] have demonstrated how several factors concerned with patient evaluation may be considered. Their concept of "available oxygen" (the amount of oxygen available for tissue perfusion) is related to (1) the cardiac output of the heart, (2) arterial oxygen saturation, (3) hemoglobin concentration, and (4) a constant of 1.34 ml/g that indicates the amount of oxygen that can combine with each gram of hemoglobin when fully saturated. The available oxygen is determined by multiplying these four factors together. If cardiac output is halved (see line two in Fig. 3-3), as it may be in a patient with myocardial damage who is further depressed by anesthetic drugs and whose

---

"Available oxygen" = Cardiac Output × Oxygen Sat. × Hemoglobin % × Constant

$$(1) \quad 1{,}000 \text{ ml/min} = 5{,}250 \text{ ml/min} \times \frac{95}{100} \times \frac{15}{100} \text{ g/100 ml} \times 1.34 \text{ ml/g}$$

$$(2) \quad 265 \text{ ml/min} = 2{,}600 \text{ ml/min} \times \frac{95}{100} \times \frac{8}{100} \text{ g/100 ml} \times 1.34 \text{ ml/g}$$

$$(3) \quad 300 \text{ ml/min} = 3{,}500 \text{ ml/min} \times \frac{64}{100} \times \frac{10}{100} \text{ g/100 ml} \times 1.34 \text{ ml/g}$$

Fig. 3-3. Examples of three cases where the "available oxygen" concept is presented.

hemoglobin is lowered to 50% of normal because of poor nutrition or occult gastrointestinal tract bleeding, then the available oxygen is reduced to one quarter of normal and is not compatible with life!

Even a moderate decrease of each one of the variables (cardiac output, hemoglobin, or oxygen saturation), when multiplied together, can produce a disastrous effect: 400 ml/min is the minimal need according to this particular schema. A little emphysema or airway obstruction superimposed on a decreased cardiac output in a moderately anemic patient may produce a severe anesthesia problem (see line three of Fig. 3-3).

Cardiac output is diminished by all anesthetic agents and depressant drugs. Congestive heart failure, aortic and mitral stenosis, hemorrhage, and constrictive pericarditis also decrease the output of the ventricles. A decrease in venomotor tone, dependent pooling, and dilation of the venous bed leads to a decrease in venous return and consequently a drop in cardiac output. Patients with cardiopulmonary disease have the greatest lung compliance in the sitting position. Dr. Samuel Levine, an internationally known Boston cardiologist, was once summoned to the bedside of a ruling dignitary in South America. After his almost 4000-mile flight he found his agitated patient in extremis and restrained in bed. He simply ordered the patient into a chair, which promptly relieved the acute symptoms, the profound effect of a simple physiologic principle.

To minimize pooling of blood in the lower limbs, a contour-type chair is advisable. The incidence of syncope associated with local anesthetic injection has been drastically reduced in dental offices with the advent of the contour chair. Another point to consider about position is the hazard of stimulation of the carotid sinus, particularly if a tight collar is worn. Some patients with advanced arteriosclerosis are easily stimulated, causing reflex bradycardia, decreased cardiac output, and resultant precipitous syncope.[16]

A number of younger patients with a history of fainting following injections are presumed to have very sensitive carotid sinus reflex mechanisms. These patients are best managed by being injected while supine, first with atropine sulfate (0.4 mg) and then with the local anesthetic. They also respond more favorably to intravenous sedation prior to local anesthetic injection.

The American Society of Anesthesiologists' system of risk classification of patients can be useful.[17] A modification follows:

Class I	Normal patients
Class II	Patients with one significant cardiopulmonary disease
Class III	Patients with two significant cardiopulmonary diseases
Class IV	Seriously ill patients requiring anesthesia, usually for emergency procedures only

Aging (older than 65 years) usually advances the patient to the next higher-risk category. It is recommended that office anesthesia be limited to patients in the first two categories. Patients who are cyanotic or dyspneic on mild exertion, show ankle edema, complain of chest pain with moderate exercise, or have other obvious stigmata of cardiopulmonary decompensation are best referred into the hospital for closer control of their medical problems and anesthetic management. Most patients manifesting cardiac dysrhythmias are best treated in close cooperation with the patient's cardiologist. In general, light intravenous sedation and local anesthesia are very effective for specific, limited dental treatment of these patients.

Pulmonary Disease

Hypoxia poses a lethal threat and oxygen must be continually provided to sustain the organism. Acute obstruction of the airway will be tolerable for only a very few minutes without producing irrevocable damage to the brain and other vital organs. Short of acute airway obstruction, other pulmonary diseases may produce serious impairment of oxygenation as well as carbon dioxide retention by interfering with the essential exchange of these gases across the pulmonary-alveolar membranes.

Acute and chronic lung infections (pneumonia, bronchitis, tuberculosis, bronchiectasis) and other disorders such as tumors and occupational diseases (silicosis) all reduce the functional capacity of the lung.

Pulmonary emphysema and bronchial asthma are two common and important lung diseases. Emphysema is typified by an increase in resistance to air flow (particularly during expiration), leading to a reduction in vital capacity and an increase in the residual volume of air trapped in the lungs. There is also obstruction of the small bronchi, in addition to a loss of elasticity and ballooning of the terminal air sacs. All these irreversible changes lead to considerably greater muscular effort and an increase in oxygen consumption. Elevated blood levels of carbon dioxide develop and cause the body to lose its normal CO_2-dependent respiratory drive. The emphysematous patient thus no longer depends on carbon dioxide to drive respiration but relies on the back-up mechanism of lowered arterial blood oxygen tension.

Further impairment of exchange by superimposed bronchitis or depression of respiration from sedatives or narcotics also poses a significant hazard. As the disease progresses and further lung areas become involved, the blood supply is shunted to more functional areas. This leads to progressive cardiac changes. In particular, the right ventricle hypertrophies and ultimately leads to cardiac failure. Emphysematous patients have shortness of breath (dyspnea) on exertion, fatigue easily, and with increasing hypoxia show cyanosis of the lips and nail beds. Dental management should be limited to emergency and palliative treatment. Nitrous oxide-oxygen sedation may allay anxiety while providing an enriched atmosphere of oxygen and reducing the work of breathing.

Caution is advised when administering oxygen to the severely emphysematous patient. Oxygen in excess of 25% to 27% may cause a respiratory arrest if the patient has lost his or her carbon dioxide drive and is functioning on oxygen-lack mechanism. The availability of a noninvasive pulse oximeter to measure oxygen saturation is an excellent aid in the management of these compromised patients.

The dyspnea of bronchial asthma is usually paroxysmal. Unlike emphysema, asthma is episodic and reversible. Dental treatment should be avoided during asthmatic attacks. The acute care of such patients includes the administration of brochodilators, fluids to improve hydration, antibiotics to control any coexisting infection, and the elimination of all respiratory irritants. Sedative drugs are useful adjuncts in the relief of asthma, but caution is essential to avoid depression of respiration.[18]

Aging and Pulmonary Function

Marshall and Miller have found that oxygen tension in the arterial tree decreases with age while arterial carbon dioxide tension remains constant.[19] Age and debility both show a decrease in blood oxygen saturation. This problem is further aggravated by cardiopulmonary disability. They found that in surgery of less than 20 minutes, arterial oxygen was not decreased below preoperative levels, but longer operations were followed by a decrease in arterial oxygen for approximately 3 hours postoperatively. Patients with pulmonary impairment not only have lower preoperative oxygen tensions but also show an even greater and more persistent fall in oxygen tension postoperatively.

These facts suggest that procedures performed under general anesthesia in older patients and those with cardiopulmonary disease should be of relatively short duration and be supplemented with more than 30% oxygen.[20] Oxygenation should be continued into the recovery period to minimize the effects of "diffusion hypoxia" and depressed ventilation.

Preoperative assessment[21] of the office patient with pulmonary disease may be done with specific questions related to exercise tolerance, cough, sputum production, smoking history, chest pain, shortness of breath, etc.

Further examination may be requested—including chest radiographs and pulmonary function studies. In the office, a breath-holding test (Sebarese's test) may be performed. The patient takes two or three deep breaths and is asked to hold the last one as long as possible. A holding time of 30 seconds or longer is normal. Less than 20 seconds indicates diminished reserve and less than 15 seconds correlates with severe compromise.

The "match test" is done by having the patient blow out a standard lighted book match held at six inches from the open mouth (without pursing the lips). Studies have shown that 85% of patients who could not blow out the match have a 1-second vital capacity or forced expiratory volume (FEV_1) below 1.6 L whereas 85% of patients who were successful in extinguishing the match have an FEV_1 greater than 1.6 L.

Neurologic Diseases

Pre-existing neurologic deficits should be noted prior to dental treatment. A past history of a cerebrovascular accident (stroke) should alert the dentist's concern for the integrity of the vascular system, and residual deficits of motor and sensory function may indicate a need to modify the anticipated treatment. Elderly patients are more susceptible to the effects of depressant medication and a very small dose may go a long way. For example, 2 mg of diazepam given intravenously may produce unconsciousness in an older patient while 20 mg may show only mild to moderate effects in the adolescent patient. Over-premedication in older patients may produce disorientation, confusion, and hypnosis rather than tranquility and cooperation.

Patients with convulsive disorders (seizures) are best managed with the aid of barbiturates or benzodiazepine sedation. Many of these patients are already taking diphenylhydantoin (Dilantin) or one of the other CNS depressant drugs, and caution is advised in the dosage of the additional premedicant agent. Diazepam is the drug of choice in the management of status epilepticus as well as sedation for other spastic disorders.

Hyperventilation by a very anxious patient may also precipitate a seizure: the carbon dioxide is blown off, and epileptogenic foci in the CNS are more likely to initiate a convulsion.

Certain other hereditary or familial diseases warrant special consideration prior to drug administration and anesthesia. Acute intermittent porphyria is an obscure disease that produces abnormal reactions, particularly when barbiturates are administered. Bizarre behavior, painful abdominal episodes, and even lower motor neuron paralysis may follow barbiturate administration. Patients with myasthenia gravis are very sensitive to nondepolarizing muscle relaxants (e.g., tubocurarine chloride) and resistant to depolarizing muscle relaxants (e.g., succinylcholine chloride). There are other patients who inherit an enzymatic deficiency and show abnormally low pseudocholinesterase levels, which cause prolonged apnea after succinylcholine administration.[22] This drug may also produce a marked, sustained rise in intraocular pressure and is dangerous to use in patients with glaucoma.[23] Patients with Down's syndrome (mongolism) respond to anticholinergic drugs (e.g., atropine) with markedly increased sensitivity, producing accentuated cardioacceleratory effects.[24]

Malignant Hyperpyrexia (Hyperthermia)

This catastrophic disorder, with a 75% mortality rate related to anesthesia, is believed to be a genetic disease of the neuromuscular apparatus. In effect, when exposed to specific anesthetic agents, muscles remain in a contracted state generating heat at an increased metabolic rate. Tachycardia is one of the constant major signs. Rapidly rising body temperature, acidosis, and muscular rigidity are prominent features. Masseteric spasm and chest wall rigidity occur early. Halothane and succinylcholine have been most frequently associated with triggering this process.

Many patients with underlying hereditary muscular dystrophies are susceptible. A muscle biopsy technique is available to help diagnose malignant hyperpyrexia by studying the muscle curve of contracture when exposed to caffeine, halothane, etc. Vigorous exercise as well as pain and anxiety may also trigger the expression of malignant hyperpyrexia. Dantrolene sodium (Dantrium), a drug used in the past to help relax muscle spasm, is now advocated to be on hand and given as early as possible to prevent the rapid evolution of this destructive process. It is recommended that 1 mg/kg be used. Side effects may include hepatic damage.

Influence of Underlying Liver and Kidney Disease

Because of the liver's primary role in the detoxification of drugs, hepatic diseases influence the selection and dosage of sedative and anesthetic agents. The most common cause of hepatic disease is alcoholism. Although faulty nutrition plays a part, the alcoholic's damage to the liver is directly related to the effect of the ethanol imbibed. Ethanol oxidation produces striking metabolic imbalances in the liver cell and leads to the accumulation of fat. The cirrhotic is a poor choice for elective dental treatment, particularly if he or she requires a general anesthetic or barbiturate sedation. Treatment should be limited to urgent or emergency problems and be accomplished with local anesthesia with adjunctive nitrous oxide-oxygen sedation or minute doses of intravenous sedative.

Similar restrictions apply to patients with advanced renal disease. The safe use of many sedative and anesthetic drugs depends upon their rapid excretion from the body. In the face of electrolyte imbalances secondary to impaired renal function the effect of these drugs is less predictable. In general, shorter-acting barbiturates are detoxified in the liver and depend less on renal excretion. There are many drugs in common use that can exacerbate kidney disease: antibiotics, narcotics, diuretics, anesthetics, and analgesics—some with more distinctive and predictable frequency.[25]

Aging per se is associated with decreased glomerular filtration by the kidney, providing increased duration of drug action and higher blood levels. Hepatic biotransformation is even more complex and often more compromised than renal clearance. Hepatic blood flow is reduced as a consequence of decreased cardiac output in the aged. Often overlooked is the real decline in muscle mass that occurs with aging as well as with the binding of drugs to protein, particularly albumen. Thus, the free fraction of the drug is available at greater levels to affect binding sites and produce a more "potent" effect.[26]

Endocrine Diseases

THYROID GLAND

Thyroid hormone serves to stimulate and regulate the metabolic activity of cells so protein synthesis and oxygen consumption are accelerated. There are a number of diseases that result in a deficiency of thyroid hormone. Endemic goiter, which produces an enlargement of the thyroid gland, is related to iodine deficiency, an element essential to the formation of thyroid hormone. When severe there are changes of skeletal development, lethargy, and deafness. The use of iodized salt prophylactically has effectively minimized the problem.

Hypothyroidism Hypothyroidism, whether caused by functional insufficiency or anatomic absence of the thyroid gland, produces marked alterations in the physical and emotional status of patients and in their ability to metabolize drugs. The hypothyroid patient may have an intolerance to cold, have dry skin, constipation, weight gain, dry sparse hair, and diminished vitality. The face appears puffy, the tongue is enlarged, and the pulse is slow and regular. Speech is slowed and mentation is retarded while the circulation is slow. Hypothyroid patients respond poorly to sedatives and narcotics with prolonged and pronounced effects to small doses. Medical treatment usually requires maintenance medication with desiccated thyroid, thyroxine, or triiodothyronine.

Hyperthyroidism (Thyrotoxicosis) Patients with hyperthyroidism have an elevated concentration of thyroid hormone. This results in an increased rate of metabolism. One form of hyperthyroidism, Graves' disease, causes prominence of the eyes. In addition to physical changes such as muscle wasting, tremor, weakness, and weight loss, there is rapid and irregular heart action that at times causes signs and symptoms of congestive heart failure. The pulse is quick and bounding and the systolic blood pressure is increased, resulting in a widening of the pulse pressure. The patient with thyrotoxicosis is a substantial risk for anesthesia and surgery. Preparation for thyroid surgery usually involves administering antithyroid medications to decrease the gland's output of thyroid hormone. In older patients, radioactive iodine is used to diminish the abnormal thyroid function.

ADRENAL GLAND

Hypoadrenalism Hypofunction or adrenocortical insufficiency (Addison's disease) poses a significant threat to the patient's survival. The development of adrenal crisis is heralded by anorexia, nausea, vomiting, headache, diarrhea, abdominal pain, dehydration, hypotension, restlessness, severe weakness, and lethargy. Coma and vascular collapse may follow. Immediate supportive care and hormonal replacement is indicated.

Most commonly, adrenal insufficiency is iatrogenic; patients receiving adrenocortical steroids over long periods lose their ability to respond to stress, surgery, and anesthesia. They must be given additional steroid medication prior to even minor surgical procedures or risk acute adrenal insufficiency. Patients with Addison's disease show increased irritability, nervousness, and emotional instability. Pigmentation usually appears early as a diffuse tanning of the skin, more marked over knees, elbows, and knuckles, and there is a bluish-black pigmentation of the mucous membranes of the mouth. In addition, these patients have hypotension and small hearts.

Hyperadrenalism (Cushing's Syndrome) Patients with excessive amounts of adrenocortical hormone, whether from an endogenous source or from corticosteroid medications, develop characteristic physical and behavioral changes. Classically, they appear with "moon facies," weight gain, muscle weakness, fat deposits over the upper back and shoulders ("buffalo hump"), and purplish skin streaks over the abdomen and hips. The skin of the face and upper chest becomes plethoric and acneiform. Osteoporosis of the spine develops. Hypertension is common and may lead to congestive heart failure. These patients are usually depressed and may become psychotic. Treatment involves removal of the tumor of the adrenal gland, or irradiation of the pituitary if a tumor is present there.

Major Mental Illnesses

Over the past two decades, the scientific literature concerning neurotransmission in the brain has exploded to expose some of the most fascinating aspects of behavior. The father of psychiatry, Sigmund Freud, predicted almost 100 years ago that one day we would find a physical basis for all mental processes. Barcas et al reported on "behavioral neurochemistry."[27] They offered a number of examples to show how neuroregulators act to adapt to environmental influences, thus bringing nature and nurture into balance.

The history of neurotransmission began with the isolation of epinephrine by Abel in 1898 and progressed to other agents such as norepinephrine, acetylcholine, dopamine, serotonin, etc., through the identification of the endorphins and enkephalins in 1964 to 1974 by Li, Reynolds, Hughes, Kosterlitz, Pert, Synder, Goldstein, Simon, and others.[28]

Since the 1950s drug treatment for mental illness has grown enormously. Presently over 25% of all prescriptions are written for psychoactive drugs. Despite beneficial influences, there are unfortunately numerous side effects of which the practitioner should be aware.

The three major disorders are generally identified as schizophrenia, depression, and mania. Current drug treatments include antipsychotics (or the so-called major tranquilizers) for schizophrenia; tricyclic antidepressants (mood elevators) and monoamine oxidase inhibitors for depression; and lithium salts for mania. Collectively, these psychoses show severe impairment of behavior and a serious inability to think coherently, to comprehend reality, or to gain insight into the abnormality. Often there are associated delusions and hallucinations. These disorders are further subdivided into organic conditions represented by delirium and dementia, quite often associated with toxic, metabolic, or neuropathologic changes, characterized by confusion, disorientation, memory disorganization, and behavioral disturbance.

The psychoses are to be differentiated from the neuroses. Neuroses usually involve less severe disturbances of behavior, are generally associated with anxiety, and exhibit signs of panic, depression, obsession, irrational fears, and compulsions. An assessment of the neurotic patient will be presented later in this chapter.

SCHIZOPHRENIA

Schizophrenia begins insidiously in childhood. The child may be somewhat withdrawn and introverted. In young adulthood, manifest symptoms of altered motor behavior, perceptual distortions, disturbed thinking, altered mood, and unusual interpersonal behavior become more apparent. These patients may show a range of motor behavior that extends from total immobility (catatonia) to frenetic and purposeless activity, often accompanied by strange mannerisms. Auditory hallucinations are quite common—the voices are often threatening and very distressing to the patient. Disturbances in thought patterns lead to distorted concept formation, bizarre speech, and paranoid delusions. Emotional responses are often absent, blunted, or inappropriate.

The incidence of schizophrenia in any population group is approximately 1%. This has remained relatively constant for the last 100 years in the United States. Such patterns of incidence imply a genetic, neurochemical etiology. Drug treatment for schizophrenia is remarkably effective in the ability to counteract hallucinations, delusional thinking, assaultiveness, severe excitement or withdrawal, and unusual behavior.

Approximately three quarters of patients are much improved by antipsychotic medications. These drugs are believed to act by blocking neuroreceptors that are stimulated by the neurotransmitter dopamine. The current hypothesis about the etiology of schizophrenia suggests that symptoms are produced as a result of an imbalance between dopamine and several other neurotransmitters, including acetylcholine, serotonin, and gamma amino butyric acid (GABA). Antipsychotic drugs that inhibit dopaminergic transmissions act to restore the proper balance. Chlorpromazine hydrochloride (Thorazine), which was first introduced in 1950 for the treatment of major psychoses, belongs to the phenothiazine group of drugs. These drugs are useful as antipsychotics, antiemetics, antinauseants, and antihistaminics and potentiate sedatives and general anesthetic agents. They produce neuroleptic effects such as decreased initiative, disinterest in the environment, decreased emotional reactivity, and a blunting of affect.

These drugs may also produce several of the characteristic changes seen with Parkinson's disease, including extrapyramidal signs. In Parkinson's these effects are caused by a deficiency of dopamine, especially in the basal ganglia leading to a predominance of cholinergic activity. Chlorpromazine also has significant alpha-adrenergic blocking effects against norepinephrine. Given intravenously, orthostatic effects may occur. The drugs also have negative inotropic effects on heart muscle. They show ECG changes such as prolongation of the QT and PR intervals with blunting of T waves and some ST depression. The antipsychotic drug thioridazine hydrochloride (Mellaril), which is a representative of the piperazine class of phenothiazines, especially causes a high incidence of T-wave changes. Prochlorperizine maleate (Compazine), another related drug, has questionable utility as an antipsychotic agent and frequently produces acute extrapyramidal reactions.

Some patients receiving antipsychotic drugs develop uncontrollable restlessness or muscle spasms in the neck, torso, or eyes. Tardive dyskinesia is a movement disorder that is distinct from the early extrapyramidal reactions in several ways: it does not respond to anticholinergic medications and is often irreversible. The dyskinesia consists of frequent repetitive involuntary movements of the lip, tongue, jaw, face, and sometimes torso and limbs. The dyskinesia is attributed to dopamine hyperactivity in the nigrostriatal pathway. Prolonged dopamine receptor blockade by the antipsychotic agents is presumed to lead to a supersensitivity of the receptors in the specific area, making them relatively more responsive to dopamine over acetylcholine activity in this region.

In 1958 haloperidol (Haldol), a butyrophenone antipsychotic agent, was introduced into clinical practice. Haldol is commonly used in the treatment of psychotic disorders. It is contraindicated in CNS depression or comatose states of any cause and in Parkinson's disease. It is used with extreme caution in combination with lithium because of the reported encephalopathic syndrome occurring in some patients on combined therapy. Patients must be warned about developing lethargy, impairment in operating machinery, or driving a motor vehicle and should also be warned about the use of alcohol together with Haldol—a combination that produces additive effects and hypotension. Other precautions are advised for patients on anticonvulsant medication: Haldol may lower the convulsive threshold. Extrapyramidal reactions occur with the administration of Haldol, and drugs such as benztropine mesylate (Cogentin) are used to counter these side effects. Cardiovascular effects include tachycardia and hypotension as well as some of the usual anticholinergic effects such as dry mouth, blurred vision, urinary retention, and increased sweating. Haloperidol is more potent than the phenothiazines such as chlorpromazine.

DEPRESSION

Psychopathologic depression is more than a transitory sadness. As a mental disorder, there are disturbances of thought patterns, motor activity, and behavior in addition to changes of mood. There are also suicidal ideas that lead to self-destructive behavior. Changes in thinking patterns lead to pessimism about the future and low self-esteem. Severely depressed patients may become psychotic, evidencing distortion of perceived reality. Physical symptoms are often a prominent part of the depression syndrome.

Classically, loss of appetite and weight are seen, as well as severe insomnia, restlessness, constipation, dry mouth, tight feelings in the chest, and aches and pains—particularly headaches, facial pains, and backaches. Many depressed people lose interest in sexual activity and depressed women often have changes in their menstrual cycles. Most depressed patients do not have a history of any other psychiatric illness.

About 20% of depressed patients have episodes of both depression and mania and are termed "bipolar." The bipolar patients alternate between depression and mania. Manic episodes are most common in younger patients whereas depression is more frequent with aging. The incidence of bipolar illness is estimated to be about 0.3% of the population. The lifetime risk of suicide with severe depression and manic depressive illness is approximately 15%. Electroconvulsive shock therapy remains the most rapid and effective treatment of severe acute depression. Electroconvulsive therapy produces decreased beta-adrenergic function (as do tricyclic antidepressants) and also dopamine receptor sensitivity.

DRUGS USED TO TREAT
DISORDERS OF MOOD

Antidepressant Medications   Tricyclic antidepressants (TCA) and monoamine oxidase (MAO) inhibitors, both introduced in 1957, are used to treat depression. Tricyclics take 2 to 4 weeks to reach their full effect and alter the symptoms of severe depression but are effective in only about 70% of patients. In most cases they cause complete remission of depressive symptoms, improve mood, restore confidence, relieve numerous physical symptoms, and eliminate suicidal thinking. Tricyclics are credited with increasing the functional activity of the neurotransmitters such as norepinephrine and serotonin. This is accomplished by a blockade of their reuptake at the receptor. The underlying hypothesis of the etiology of depressive states is that depression is caused by a functional underactivity or deficiency of these neurotransmitters. Mania on the other hand, is associated with their functional hyperactivity. Tricyclics such as imipramine hydrochloride (Tofranil) block the reuptake of serotonin and control psychomotor agitation, whereas amitriptyline hydrochloride (Elavil) inhibits uptake of norepinephrine and promotes psychomotor activation.

Tricyclic antidepressants are known to potentiate the effects of directly acting sympathomimetic amines such as tyramine, which is taken up by sympathetic neurons to effect the release of norepinephrine. This leads to an increased tendency for dysrhythmias. Tricyclics also cause a decrease in blood pressure and obtund certain postural and cardiovascular reflexes. Both myocardial infarction and congestive heart failure have been attributed to imipramine. The electrocardiograph shows flattening and inversion of T waves, representing a quinidine-like myocardial depressant effect. The half-life of the drug given orally is 20 hours, and the agent takes approximately a week to clear.

The tricyclics also show considerable anticholinergic effect. Symptoms such as blurred vision, dry mouth, constipation, and urinary retention are seen. The latter is especially noted to occur with amitriptyline. In addition, the patient may complain of a metallic taste, epigastric distress, and paradoxically, excessive sweating. Imipramine may also precipitate manic excitement and delirium in about 10% of patients. Children appear to be particularly vulnerable to the cardiotoxic and seizure-inducing effects of high doses of tricyclics.

The tricyclic antidepressants are potentiated by neuroleptic drugs and certain steroids, including oral contraceptives. Barbiturates, which increase microsomal enzyme function, result in a decreased effect of tricyclics. Tricyclics also potentiate alcohol and other sedatives as well as blocking guanethidine effect centrally, used to decrease blood pressure. The antidepressant tricyclics have also been used for the management of chronic pain, particularly atypical facial pain, and have shown a high degree of success, especially when the complaint is a "depressive equivalent." Fluoextine hydrochloride (Prozac), a relatively new antidepressant, interferes with uptake of serotonin but not of norepinephrine. It is widely used.

Monoamine Oxidase Inhibitors Monoamine oxidase (MAO) inhibitors have been cut back in their use in favor of tricyclic antidepressants because of the high incidence of untoward side effects. There are two types of MAO inhibitors recognized: type A deaminates serotonin and type B deaminates dopamine and phenylethylamine (PEA). In the presence of MAO inhibitors, biogenic amines are not deaminated but remain active and prolong and intensify the effect of transmitters such as dopamine and serotonin. Amino inhibitors also interfere with the detoxification of other drugs and prolong and intensify the central depressant effects of general anesthetics, sedatives, antihistamines, alcohol, analgesics, anticholinergics, and antidepressants such as imipramine and amitriptyline. Serious hypertension may occur with meperidine, which is related to the release of serotonin. A hypertensive crises secondary to tyramine in various foods is occasionally seen when inhibition of MAO type A occurs. This is caused by a massive release of norepinephrine from tyramine-rich foods.

An increased level of MAO type B is found in presenile dementia (Alzheimer's disease and Huntington's disease).[29] Recently, patients with Alzheimer's disease have been shown to have a significantly decreased concentration of choline acetyltransferase, the enzyme that makes the neurotransmitter acetylcholine.[30]

DRUGS USED TO TREAT MANIA

Lithium is used in the treatment of mania. In normal man it shows no psychotropic effects. Although its mechanism of action is unknown, lithium carbonate corrects sleeplessness in the manic patient. It has a low margin of safety, requiring divided daily doses. With depletion of sodium, as may occur with patients taking diuretics, high and toxic levels of lithium may be produced. Lithium intoxication is usually seen as vomiting, profuse diarrhea, ataxia, coma, and convulsions with cardiac arrhythmias and hypotension. Lithium decreases the pressure response to norepinephrine. Its effects on the cardiovascular system appear as depression of T waves while toxic doses widen the QRS complex.

DRUGS USED TO TREAT ANXIETY

In 1977, specific CNS receptors were identified for the benzodiazepines with about 70% of the binding occurring in the synaptic membrane. The distribution of these stereospecific receptors is highest in the cerebral cortex, followed by the hypothalamus, cerebellum, corpus striatum, and medulla. This parallels the receptors of GABA but they are not identical.

Benzodiazepines potentiate the inhibitory effect of GABA and other inhibitory transmitters in the CNS. GABA is made by decarboxylation of glutamic acid. Neurons that generate GABA also influence the activity of other neurons that secrete dopamine or serotonin. Anesthetics tend to increase the concentration of GABA. The counterpart to GABA in the brain appears to be the simplest amino acid, glycine, which has major inhibitory transmitter action in the spinal cord and brain system.[31]

An unusual property of the benzodiazepine receptors is their apparent lack of affinity for any of the known neurotransmitters or any of the known agonists. The use of a new drug, RO15-1788, by Geller et al[32] was shown to be a specific benzodiazepine antagonist. It was marketed under the name of Flumazenil in 1991. Benzodiazepines may influence postsynaptic phenomena at the GABA synapses. They potentiate the effects of GABA. Data also suggest that benzodiazepines facilitate the action of GABA in its anticonvulsant effects.

The sedative and antianxiety effects of benzodiazepines can be distinguished from their muscle relaxant effects. The antianxiety properties are distinguished from the sedative properties by different dose-response relationships. This has important implications for the practice of pain and anxiety control in dentistry. Antianxiety doses of benzodiazepines do not influence GABA metabolism or release GABA from presynaptic nerve terminals. (Benzodiazepines have a glycinemimetic effect on the spinal cord and brainstem.) Another theory for the antianxiety effect of benzodiazepines suggests that these agents decrease the activity of serotonin and acetylcholine by promoting GABA-mediated inhibition of serotonin-mediated transmission.

On cardiovascular and respiratory systems, intravenous diazepam in 5- to 10-ml doses causes slight decrease in respiration, blood pressure, and left ventricular stroke work. It also causes some increase in heart rate and decrease in cardiac output. The effects overall are rather mild. In recent study of Jordan et al 15-mg doses of diazepam showed respiratory depression that could be relieved by large doses of naloxone.[33]

Benzodiazepines have minimal pharmacologic interactions with other drugs except for MAO inhibitors. Extreme care is urged in the administration of benzodiazepines to elderly or ill patients and those with limited pulmonary-cardiac reserve. Concomitant use of barbiturates and other CNS depressants increases depression while increasing the risk of apnea. It is recommended that when diazepam is used with a narcotic analgesic the dosage of narcotics be reduced by at least one third and administered in small increments. Diazepam should not be administered to patients in shock, in a coma, or with depression of vital signs.

The *Medical Letter* (February 1981)[34] suggests that stopping a long-acting drug such as diazepam may precipitate a withdrawal psychosis that then may be easily misdiagnosed as physiologic reactions to hospitalization or to an operation. It has also been pointed out that the drug cimetidine (Tagamet), when used along with diazepam results in a higher blood level of the tranquilizer. Tagamet inhibits the hepatic microsomal enzymes that metabolize diazepam, and when these drugs are used together the plasma diazepam level is increased by one third.[35]

The administration of diazepam to patients in the extremes of age shows a three to four times longer half-life. The presence of hepatic disease also increases the half-life two to five times. Occasionally, overdose of diazepam leads to an increase in hostility and irritability or paradoxically to an increase in anxiety. Diazepam is very effective in relieving spasticity in patients with cerebral palsy and is also used extensively in cardioversion and in control of acute seizure disorders.

New developments in the field of brain neurochemistry are defining some of the mechanisms that affect human behavior. These serve several purposes: they offer greater promise for the future correction of deviant patterns of perception, thought, and action; they teach us more about the potential interactions of anesthetics and psychoactive drugs; and perhaps of even broader significance, they enable us to understand some of the physical and mental states that for ages have threatened laymen and professional alike. Somehow it is easier to relate to patients with aberrant behavior if there is a recognized physical basis for the aberration. This lessens one's own fear of loss of control and improves predictability of patient response.

The Medical and Personal History

History taking is a science and an art. Recognition of the interrelationship between the details of the medical history and the patient's personal history provides important insights into how the patient has reacted to current treatment. What is said in response to questions is as important as the *way* in which it is said, as well as what is omitted.

All doctors are trained to take a medical history. They have spent many hours at bedside and chairside asking pertinent questions to help them evaluate the patient's illness and history. Their primary interest in such questioning is to define the course of the disease or defect and then to analyze that patient's physical status in anticipation of treatment. However, the "art" of history taking involves much more—it is an attempt to develop a more comprehensive picture of the whole person and to evaluate his or her response to our treatment.

The art of history taking is grounded in the doctor-patient relationship. It is based on the ancient but prevailing human need to be helped in a time of "dis-ease." This relationship is a two-way interaction. We learn to fulfill the role of doctor through many years of study, but study alone does not make an empathetic or compassionate healer. In fact, there are data to show that students who initially select medicine or dentistry become more callous and indifferent to patients as one of the side effects of their professional education.

Nevertheless, the high ideals that determined the doctor's choice of career are in evidence, and most doctors carry out their responsibilities to their patients with dedication. Much of this compassion and dedication is learned on the basis of identification with one's mentors; wise teachers recognize their special responsibility to set good examples because of this fact. Because the doctor's relationship to his or her patient is so crucial to the success of treatment and the art of history taking is germinal in this relationship, this art will be explored in depth.

Just as we ask about the medical history, we should develop an appreciation for what we shall call the "personal history." The modern dentist deals with considerably more than the patient who is impelled by pain and swelling to seek emergency relief. Especially in the areas of reconstructive treatment and maxillofacial-orthognathic surgery, one is impressed with the need to gain important insights into the patient's behavior and motivation. Although patients manage to chew and grow despite severe malocclusions, they become emotionally marred by the facial deformity especially when they do not have any hope of changing their perceived ugliness. Helping the patient surgically, even when the operation is successfull anatomically, may not be enough to repair the years of psychologic damage. In this instance, the personal history provides a tool for assessment of the extent of the damage and is one of the keys to dealing with these problems concurrently.

One of the primary aims in taking a personal history is to help establish the rapport that precedes successful treatment. This rapport is essential for many reasons. One is the therapeutic effect of the patient's subjective feeling of the doctor's concern and interest. Another is prevention of a breakdown of the doctor-patient relationship that can lead to medico-legal problems. Patterns of behavior elicited in the personal history can alert the doctor to potential problems. Many doctors who have a well-functioning professional relationship avoid vindictive suits and complaints even when the surgical result is far from satisfactory. The patients recognize that they have been treated humanely, to the best of the doctor's ability, and that they have not been belittled or abandoned. In this regard, the image of the old-time comforting "Doc" who did the best he could with limited medications and methods is never associated with the bitterness one finds in practice today. Sixty-four percent of all patients criticize their doctors for a lack of warmth. They may be satisfied with the quality of care but dislike the way it is given. Alarmingly, 70% of the population approves of the use of nonmedical healers, including chiropractors and quacks.[36] Because of their anger with their doctors, many patients fail to pay their bills. Malpractice suits are often dramatic symptoms of the breakdown in the doctor-patient relationship. It is fair to say that the old-time "Doc" dispensed concern and support in large measures, instead of quick, hollow-sounding reassurance or the hastily prescribed placebo.

What are some of the other reasons for taking a personal history? Very often even in our society, dentists function as primary physicians. By virtue of their extensive training, not only in problems of the head and neck but in other systemic disorders as well, they are the first to see a neglected hypertensive patient or a patient with any constellation of systemic complaints, some of which have oral components. By taking a personal history, the dentist gains additional insights into the overall health of the patient and is better able to manage the oral problem.

There is still another reason to take a personal history. Sometimes the oral complaints are exacerbated by underlying psychologic difficulties. Without appreciating the psychologic contribution to the symptoms, the doctor may overtreat medically or misdiagnose the condition. For example, emotional immaturity will often become manifest in patients who make unusual and unrealistic demands. This relates to their inability to accept the recommended treatment as well as to their inability to cope with the side effects and after effects of treatment. The cooperation of patients may be significantly undermined.

Just as we acquire specific education to learn the methods and techniques of dentistry, so also do we need to learn the techniques involved in eliciting a pertinent personal history. Much personal information is gained during the direct medical history taking. We listen not only for

factual answers but also to the tone and timing of the responses. We observe various body movements and postural changes. Writers have enlarged on this area of "body language" primarily in the social setting.

We are aware of the patient who avoids our gaze and looks away when answering questions. We note the apprehension reflected in a tense and rigid posture: gripping the armrests of the chair, crossing and uncrossing legs, or shifting uncomfortably to adjust the headrest. Many of these are indicative of anxiety, which spans the spectrum from normal to neurotic to psychotic anxiety.

We should be more aware of our own reactions to what the patient is saying and to his or her movements. Your own inner feedback provides important information that can help you respond more appropriately to the patient. An experienced practitioner will intuitively respond in a more appropriate manner, realizing that a patient's belligerence may be masking fear rather than being an intentional challenge to the doctor. The patient's answers may be direct, tangential and evasive, or brief and inappropriate.

If you desire more information after the exchange of medical history questions, you may want to encourage this by saying, "Is there anything else you would like to ask or tell me about yourself?" Or, "Is there anything we haven't discussed that you feel is important that I should know?" It may also be helpful to focus this part of the interview toward the patient's interactions with family, friends, and school or work experiences.

Most dentists are reluctant to get involved in this type of discussion; they feel uncomfortable and worry about "how deep to go," which is often the projection of the doctor's feelings rather than the patient's. This reluctance can be helped by learning when and how to cut off further discussion. An indication that you have gone too deep might be when the patient's defenses are challenged, such as when you ask the same question repeatedly, in spite of evidence that the patient is uncomfortable and does not want to discuss it. The patient may also feel challenged if the doctor verbalizes his or her hasty interpretation of these defenses. Comments on the patient's psychologic processes may be better left unspoken.

Only an occasional patient will voluntarily go further than he or she feels comfortable with. Such a situation is easily handled by accepting or acknowledging the patient's problem rather than by offering empty reassurances that are immediately perceived as denying the patient's concerns. It is important to acknowledge the patient's problem and to recommend a means of dealing with it, which may take the form of consultation with the patient's physician, pediatrician, or psychiatrist. The oft-heard phrase "Don't worry" is useless and is usually interpreted to mean "Don't bother me with your problems." It is therefore important not to confront the manner in which the patient copes. Don't challenge the patient's defenses—this will usually lead to more distress on the part of the patient and to more inappropriate behavior. When you find yourself trying to deny the patient's method of coping, you will realize that you are going too far. It is time to redirect or cut off this line of approach.

CASE REPORT

An attractive 13-year-old girl was referred to the office because of a huge cyst of the mandible that histologically proved to be a plexiform ameloblastoma. In subsequent discussion with the child and her mother, a treatment plan involving hemimandibulectomy and immediate bone grafting was presented. The child was invited to ask questions but remained passive and deferred to her mother. At a later appointment, a rather comprehensive presentation about hospitalization, anesthesia, and functional, anatomic, and esthetic considerations was discussed. Again the child asked only a few superficial questions but the mother indicated that the girl was upset.

Preoperatively the patient was referred to a psychiatrist for consultation. He quickly elicited her tremendous fear and concern about the operation, and in particular, her fantasy of not being able to walk or dance, secondary to the iliac bone graft. It was apparent that her anxiety had caused her to block out major areas of the planning discussions. The psychiatrist and oral surgeon conferred and, at a second appointment, the psychiatrist was able to provide more realistic and reassuring support. The operation and hospitalization were successful and the child rapidly regained her normal effective manner of relating to friends, family, and doctors. She was very cooperative throughout and had a gratifying surgical result.

Because this was an elective procedure, we believed that it was important to prepare this patient optimally rather than rushing into surgery. The same maxim holds true with almost all of our maxillofacial-orthognathic surgical patients. One measure of success has been the very high rate of prolonged follow-up care.

Assessment of the Neurotic Patient

Who is neurotic? What are the boundaries of this ill-defined designation? Or better still, how can we elicit this necessary information to help us appropriately manage these patients and their problems? Classically, neurosis is defined as a "functional nervous disease or one which is dependent upon no evident lesion . . . a peculiar state of tension or irritability . . . any form of nervousness."[37] The medical and personal histories can be very helpful determining when patients require special consideration because of neuroses. Are we dealing with a confused, disoriented patient who has an organic brain syndrome? Is this secondary to senility, or is it related to metabolic disease such as the diabetic who is hypoglycemic, the uremic patient or the chronic alcoholic with brain damage, or the patient with head trauma with a concussion syndrome or a subdural hematoma? What can we discern about the patient's mood and affect? Are we talking to a depressed patient who uses few words, and who speaks slowly and haltingly? Are we dealing with an "uptight" patient who is hostile or withdrawn and uncooperative?

What are some of the mechanisms that potentially troublesome patients use? Seduction by flattery is one of the primary techniques. The trap is baited by the patient who flatters the doctor into assuming a position he may not be able to fulfill. Criticism of other doctors is another warning sign of the troublesome patient. Usually this criticism is used in conjunction with flattery. It should be immediately apparent to the doctor that he is about to join the list of those criticized.

Other indicators of the potentially troublesome patient are gleaned from the history and include such disclosures as frequent changes of physicians or dentists because of dissatisfaction; anger over charges by doctors and hospitals; evidences of past uncooperativeness in treatment plans; accusation against doctors for failing to do enough for family, friends, or self during previous illnesses; and remarks of distrust of the skill and honesty of the profession.

Why is it so important to gain this information by history taking and observing the behavior of the patient? Because the life-styles of troublesome patients are so consistent and their relationship to you will tend to follow previous trends. The best indicator of a troublesome patient comes from within yourself. "It is the symptom which makes the doctor begin to feel that he ought to be or act like the protecting, truth-concealing, responsibility-taking, or fatherly person that his patient flatteringly implies he is."[38]

There are some consulting dental practitioners who make routine use of a patient aptitude test such as the Cornell Medical Index* or the Minnesota Multiphasic Personality Inventory.+ These tests are helpful when dealing with patients who have chronic facial or temporomandibular joint pain. These are simple to administer and score and can be a very informative medical and psychologic profile. A score above a certain level alerts the practitioner to the likelihood of significant psychologic difficulty that would directly affect the treatment. These tests

---

*Cornell Medical Index, available from Cornell University Medical College, 1300 York Avenue, New York, NY 10021.

+Minnesota Multiphasic Personality Inventory, available from Psychological Corp., 757 Third Avenue., New York, NY 10017.

are aids and do not obviate the need to discuss personal history with the patient. They are analogous to medical questionnaires that serve as aids in eliciting further important information.[39] Following are representative questions from these types of tests.

Identifying data (age, sex . . .)

Chief complaint

History of present illness

Past medical history

Review of symptoms

Understanding about illness ("What's your understanding of what's wrong?")

Current life situations:

Family and friends (quality of relationships)

Present occupation and economic status (attitude toward work)

Leisure activities ("What do you do for fun?")

Social and community commitments

Personal characteristics and pattern of living (cultural background, manner of coping with stress, typical day)

Past development

Childhood and adolescence

Educational and occupational history

Marital and family history

Description of patient (general appearance, cooperativeness)

Mental status (as indicated)

What is the psychosocial impact of this operation or illness?

Predisposing Factors

As a general rule, patients who have experienced illness from early childhood because of congenital, developmental, metabolic, or severe infectious diseases with lasting sequelae have significant behavioral changes.

We cite a recent case of an 18-year-old boy with a limp secondary to a congenital hip defect, who sustained a fracture of the jaw that required admission to the hospital for an open reduction. He had been "beat up by three friends." Four months previously, he had undergone a closed reduction of his mandibular fracture after also being "beat up." His arch bars were still in place because he had failed to keep his postoperative appointments. The boy was withdrawn and uncommunicative, refusing to talk with any of his nurses, doctors, social worker, or psychiatrist. Two days postoperatively, he left the hospital against medical advice and again failed to keep his postoperative appointments. This is a rather stark example of deviant behavior bordering on distinct self-destructive, suicidal tendencies, including his role in the provocation of fights that led to repeated injuries. We may assume that he had a very poor self-image, starting with his congenital hip deformity.

The juvenile diabetic or the hemophilic youngster may show evidence of self-destructiveness. Growing up with a major handicap magnifies feelings of inadequacy, worthlessness, and guilt. The guilt is often attributed to a belief by the child that he or she has done something wrong and is therefore being punished with illness or disability. If he or she is different from other children, then he or she must be "bad" and deserving of punishment. This kind of reasoning can be seen in the hemophiliac who denies his past history in order to have the dentist extract his sore tooth. It is experienced in the juvenile diabetic who ignores his dietary limitations and his insulin regimen with resultant episodes of diabetic acidosis. It is not too uncommon to find unhappy adolescents who drink excessively or take addicting drugs. Certainly these patients justify careful evaluation before oral surgical treatment is undertaken.

Varying degrees of self-destructiveness are readily seen in many patients. Perhaps the most common example is the widespread incidence of advanced dental neglect where even well-educated patients from higher socioeconomic groups have extensive carious lesions and periodontal breakdown and do not actively seek regular treatment and preventive care.

Previous responses to early illness and disability and the patient's compliance with treatment largely influence and indicate future responses. We continue to emphasize this interaction of the patient's emotional responses and his physical disease. The personality will often determine the way in which one reacts to physical disease. The middle-aged patient who has sustained a myocardial infarction often suffers more from the emotional reaction to the catastrophe than to the physical scar in the heart muscle. Typically, there is confusion, anger, denial of imposed limitation, and an effort to prove his or her continuing competence.[39] Often the patient's actions threaten his or her very survival. The basis of these apparent inappropriate reactions is probably grounded in a long-standing unconscious sense of insecurity. As long as he or she functioned in the usual routine, this was masked. But with a crumbling of defenses secondary to significant physical impairment, the ability to cope and respond was severely compromised.

It is important to understand the dynamics of these reactions so that we can help a patient develop more appropriate defenses to deal with these insecurities at this crucial time. Specifically, patients after myocardial infarction are encouraged to see their progress and improvement as well as to feel rewarded for their ability to cope in spite of their frightening experience. We help these patients re-establish a sense of adequacy in a way that does not further jeopardize their lives. For example, allowing himself to be passive and in bed is a sign of great strength and adequacy that should be acknowledged: "You're doing fine; you're showing an awful lot of strength in following the doctor's recommendation to take it easy." A similar approach is taken for surgical patients who have sustained injuries or undergone extensive elective surgery that require a certain pattern of passivity and cooperation.[39]

Most persons react to their anticipated surgical experience with evidence of increased endogenous catecholamines. For the patient with an irritable cardiac conduction system, this can lead to abnormalities of rate and rhythm[40] as well as precipitating congestive failure in a patient whose myocardium cannot respond with an appropriate cardiac output demanded by an increase in heart rate. These patients often require careful monitoring, light pharmacologic sedation, and, above all, understanding and considerable emotional support for their total problem. Hyperventilation, angina, and acute anxiety attacks are not infrequent.

With pulmonary problems two major areas of concern include asthmatic and emphysematous patients. Current thinking provides a reformulation of the cause of asthma. It is a disease that requires a predisposition of the bronchiolar substrate, which may then react adversely to allergy, infection, or psychologic stress. Usual treatment is directed to the control of infection and of allergy as well as supportive care with bronchodilating drugs. In the absence of infection and allergy, asthmatic patients undergoing anesthesia and oral surgery require special care. Sometimes maintenance steroid therapy is increased to carry the patient through this stress. More often, management can be successful by provision of more emotional support.

Recently, a 17-year-old severely asthmatic girl underwent surgery for an impaction without exacerbation of her disease. Management began with the mother's initial phone call, which provided adequate time to vent her anxieties about her daughter's condition. The oral surgeon then scheduled a consultation visit for examination, radiographs, and history taking. The girl was extremely apprehensive and shy. A program of treatment was discussed that allowed the girl to decide whether she would have general anesthesia or conscious intravenous sedation. She preferred to be awake but sedated and voiced her deep concern about avoiding a facial or nasal mask. She was anxious about anything over her nose or mouth that might affect her breathing. The patient was encouraged to talk and take an active part in this situation rather than allow her mother to dominate and direct the treatment.

Typical of many asthmatic patients, she was a frightened and dependent person in need of considerable emotional support. Giving her an opportunity to vent her concerns was an important part of the successful management and led to realistic reassurances that the surgeon was aware of her problems and was prepared to help her handle any difficulties. Similarly, emphyse-

matous patients need additional reassurance to minimize stress and decrease the likelihood of further ventilatory demand and hypoxia. In addition, one should be cautious about the use of oxygen in excess of 24% to 27% if the compromised patient is functioning on oxygen chemoreceptor drive. Excess oxygen can precipitate apnea and ventilatory arrest. Although mild sedation is helpful, narcotics and deep sedation are contraindicated in the emphysematous patient.

Finally, let us turn the mirror around and look at the doctor. Because the doctor-patient relationship is really an important two-way process, what are some of the personality characteristics the doctor may contribute?

We should recognize that there are certain defenses that new doctors use. The training of most oral surgeons takes place in busy municipal hospitals and often involves indigent patients who are seen for emergency or episodic care. The oral surgery resident does not have to be concerned about adequacy of patient numbers. These patients frequently have nowhere else to go and must submit to this clinic. This can lead to what we would term "city hospital exodontia"—a depersonalized and frenetic atmosphere where forceps flash and teeth and tissues fly.

Compare this to the young oral surgical graduate who is developing his or her own practice and must depend for his or her successful growth on interpersonal relationships with patients and referring doctors. Dr. Smith, who has to make that bridge for Mrs. Jones, will not be tolerant of a destroyed buccal plate. Nor will he appreciate Mrs. Jones' report of how indifferently she was treated, including the prolonged, painful follow-up treatments. The young surgeon quickly learns surgical finesse and strives to improve the management of patients. More confidence is developed which is reflected in a calm demeanor and a businesslike office. The surgeon learns to encourage patients to ventilate their fears and anxieties and thereby allow for a reduction of their concerns.

From my early days of office visiting, I recall a very successful oral surgeon who had developed the ability to produce what we would call "instant" rapport. I watched as a very apprehensive 30-year-old woman was seated and prepared for a short general anesthetic and the removal of two teeth. The surgeon entered the room, placed a hand gently on the patient's shoulder, introduced himself, and greeted the woman. Instant, visible, and audible relief was expressed by the patient. Her tense posture relaxed, she felt his calm, confident manner and, after a few more moments, was much more amenable to the anticipated anesthesia and surgery. He had learned how to approach anxious patients and to help them relax and feel more assured of his ability. He presented himself as a person exuding confidence and also recognized the woman as a person in need of support.

Patients cannot readily appreciate the doctor's technical skills but they can readily grasp those interpersonal and professional interchanges that make them feel comfortable and confident.

Neurotic dentists, like neurotic patients, need help and better insight into their self-sabotaging behavior. There are several important indications of such disruptive and destructive behavior. One of the most glaring is for a male dentist to treat a female patient, especially one who is under nitrous oxide or other mind-altering drugs, in the absence of a third person. Such behavior may provoke accusations of sexual exploitation, which are almost impossible to refute.

Another is the concern by the practitioner who cannot discern any objective findings despite careful examination and is loath to tell the patient that the examination is negative and that further examination or consultation may be required if symptoms persist. Instead, the dentist invokes that currently popular disease known as "TMJ" and commits the patient to a variety of iatrogenic insults. Or he or she proceeds with endodontic treatment or extraction in the absence of objective criteria. The dentist is obviously unaware of "Trieger's dictum," which is "You cannot cure with dental treatment that which is not dental disease." Many a patient with tic douloureux or atypical facial pain has been inappropriately treated and falls into this category. The urge to "do something" for the chronic pain patient or the patient with "burning tongue" is fraught with real hazard, especially for the insecure dentist. Doing something constructive may also take the form of careful and considerate attention to history and physical examination rather than rushing to do some irreversible procedure.

Aberrant behavior by the practitioner is receiving more attention. Hospital administrators and colleagues on the attending staff are legally enjoined to report individuals who are impaired through the use of alcohol or drugs, and even mental and physical infirmities that affect their management of patients. Professional standards are being raised and strictures applied. In most instances this type of policing action is accompanied by significant offers of help for the identified practitioner. It would obviously be far better if such doctors were able to recognize their problems earlier and avoid jeopardizing their productive careers. Perhaps we who are professionally trained in hospital settings to view the whole person could take a more active and objective role in helping ourselves and our colleagues.

Summary

While careful pretreatment medical evaluation is necessary for every patient, it is particularly critical for those patients being considered for adjunctive medications. An assessment of each individual's physical condition must consider the primacy of the cardiovascular status because many other factors bear on this common denominator. The presence or absence of congenital heart defects, coronary artery disease, dysrhythmia, anemia, diseases of the lungs, hypertension, diabetes, obesity, and neurologic, hepatic, renal, and endocrine system disorders must be assessed prior to effective and safe treatment. Specific allergies or medications being taken should be elicited by a careful medical history review.

It is also important when obtaining a history to evaluate the patient's mental status. A small but significant number of patients are overtly psychotic and are receiving drugs that distinctly alter mentation and behavior but also precipitate adverse drug effects and adverse drug interactions. A larger number of patients exhibit a wide variety of neurotic symptoms that may masquerade as severe physical impairments. It is appropriate to expand the assessment of patients to gain insights into their previous responses to illness, disabilities, and treatments and to seek further consultation with their physicians, neurologists, or psychiatrists when suspicion is raised and more information and guidance are needed.

Only after such an evaluation should the dentist proceed with extensive or irreversible treatment. It is advisable to limit office treatment to patients who are in good general health or whose disease status is well controlled. Those patients who pose greater risk should be referred to a hospital for more extensive supervision and care.

References

1. Guyton AC: Regulation of cardiac output, *N Engl J Med* 277(15): 805-812, 1967.
2. Abramowitz M: *Med Letter Drugs Ther* 31:109, 1989.
3. Sadowsky D, Kunzel C: Clinician compliance and the prevention of bacterial endocarditis, *J Am Dent Assoc* 109:425-428, 1984.
4. Mason DT et al: Physiologic approach to the treatment of angina pectoris, *N Engl J Med* 281 (22):1225-1228, 1969.
5. Steen PA, Tinker JH, Tarhan S: Myocardial reinfarction after anesthesia and surgery, *J Am Med Assoc* 239:2556-2570, 1978.
6. Abramowitz M: Nifedipine for angina pectoris, *Med Lett Drugs Ther* 24:39-40, 1982.
7. Cahill GF, McDevitt HO: Insulin dependent diabetes mellitus: the inital lesion, *N Engl J Med* 304 (24):1454-1464, 1981.
8. Raskin P et al: The effect of diabetic control on the width of skeletal muscle capillary basement membrane in patients with type I diabetes mellitus, *N Engl J Med* 309 (25):1546-1550, 1983.
9. Schade DS, Easton RP: Insulin delivery: how, when and where, *N Engl J Med* 312:17, 1985.
10. Kannel WB et al: Role of blood pressure in the development of congestive heart failure, *N Engl J Med* 287 (16):781-787, 1972.
11. Amer MS: Cyclic adenosine monophosphate and hypertension in rats, *Science* 182:179-809, 1973.
12. Marx JL: Natriuretic hormone linked to hypertension, *Science* 212: 1255-1257, 1981.
13. McCarron DA et al: Blood pressure and nutrient intake in the United States, *Science* 224: 1392-1398, 1984.
14. Kannel WB et al: Epidemiologic features of chronic atrial fibrillation, *N Engl J Med* 306 (17):1018-1022, 1982.
15. Nunn JF, Freeman J: Problems of oxygenation and oxygen transport during hemorrhage, *Anesthesiology* 19(1):120-121; 19(2):206-216, 1964.
16. Allen GD: *Dental anesthesia and analgesia,* ed 3, Baltimore, 1984, Williams & Wilkins.
17. American Society of Anesthesiologists: New classification of physical status, *Anesthesiology* 24:111, 1963.
18. McKaba DG: Management of the non-hospitalized asthmatic patient, *Curr Conc Allerg Clin Immunol* 2 (2):1-6, 1973.
19. Marshall BE, Miller RA: Some factors influencing postoperative hypoxemia, *Anesthesiology* 20(4):408-427, 1965.
20. Lewin I et al: Physical class and physiologic status in prediction of operative mortality in aged sick, *Ann Surg* 174:217-231, 1971.
21. Goldsmith D, Trieger N: Pulmonary assessment in the ambulatory patient, *J Oral Surg* 38:771-773, 1980.
22. Harmel MH: Medical drug therapy and anesthesia, *Proc Int Med* 25(10): 291-293, 1965.
23. American Medical Association: *AMA Drug Evaluations,* ed 1, Chicago, 1971, American Medical Association.
24. Harris WS, Goodman RM: Hyper-reactivity to atropine in Down's syndrome, *N Engl J Med* 279(8):407-409, 1968.
25. Martin EW et al: *Hazards of medicine,* Philadelphia, 1971, JB Lippincott.
26. Greenblatt DJ, Sellers EM, Shader RI: Drug therapy: drug deposition in old age, *N Engl J Med* 306(18):1081-1088.
27. Barcas JD et al: Behavioral neurochemistry: neuroregulators and behavioral states, *Science* 200:964-973, 1978.
28. Trieger N: Newer neurotransmitters in pain control, *Anesth Prog* 26:66-71, 1979.
29. Mann JJ et al: Mental symptoms in Huntington's disease and a possible primary aminergic neuron lesion, *Science* 208: 1369-1371, 1980.

30. Robinson A: Clues to the cause of senile dementia, *Science* 211:1032-1033, 1981.

31. Richter JJ: Current theories about the mechanisms of benzodiazepines and neuroleptic drugs (medical intelligence), *Anesthesia* 54:66-72, 1981.

32. Geller E et al: The use of RO 15-1788: a benzodiazepine antagonist in the diagnosis and treatment of benzodiazepine overdose, *Anesthesiology* 61(3A):A135, 1984.

33. Jordan C et al: Respiratory depression following diazepam. Reversed with high-dose naloxone, *Anesthesiology* 53:293-298, 1980.

34. Abramowicz M: Drugs that cause psychiatric symptoms, *Med Lett* 23:3, 1981.

35. Klotz U, Reimann I: Delayed clearance of diazepam due to cimetidine, *N Engl J Med* 302:1012-1014, 1980.

36. Koss E: What people think of their medical services, *Am J Pub Health* 45:1551, 1955.

37. *Stedman's Medical Dictionary,* ed 24, Baltimore, 1982, Williams & Wilkins, p 949.

38. Blum RH: *The management of the doctor-patient relationship,* New York, 1960, McGraw Hill.

39. Strain JJ, Grossman S: *A primer of liaison psychiatry,* New York, 1976, Appleton-Century Crofts.

40. Lown B, Verrier RL: Neural activity and ventricular fibrillation, *N Engl J Med* 294:1165, 1976.

4

New Approaches to Local Anesthesia

The use of local anesthesia to obtund painful stimuli in dentistry and other surgical specialties has been one of the marvels of the twentieth century. It has made possible the great range of surgical and therapeutic services provided by dentists and surgeons around the world. Local anesthesia surely must be regarded as one of the most important cornerstones of pain control. If dentists were to be suddenly deprived of local anesthetics, their services would literally grind to a halt.

Before discussing how and why local anesthetic agents produce their effects, pragmatic practitioners and students will prefer to review the techniques and anatomic considerations for producing regional anesthesia in dentistry. Anatomically we are concerned almost exclusively with the maxillary and mandibular division of the fifth cranial nerve, the trigeminal. Several intraoral injection techniques will be described, beginning with more proximal nerve blocks and progressing to more peripheral sites.

Maxillary Nerve Block

With one well-placed injection, the entire hemimaxilla may be anesthetized. This particular technique is not widely taught or practiced, although it is a remarkably effective nerve block when extensive treatment is planned. Perhaps we are at a time comparable to where we were 50 years ago, when most dental schools did not teach mandibular block anesthesia but instead relied upon a variety of peripheral infiltrations and pericemental injections. Admittedly, the maxillary cortical bone is not as thick as that of the mandible, and the distributions of the posterior, middle, and anterior superior alveolar branches of the maxillary nerve are more super-

ficial than the inferior alveolar nerve, which lies deep within the body of the mandible. Nevertheless, the maxillary nerve block has a decided advantage over multiple buccal, labial, and palatal injections, which are obviated by an effective single more proximal block of the nerve trunk. There are two basic techniques advocated.

THE GREATER PALATINE FORAMEN INJECTION

This technique is performed with the use of a 25-gauge needle and aspirating syringe. This foramen is situated in the posterior palate between the second and third molars (Fig. 4-1), about 1 cm from the palatal gingival margin toward the midline of the palate. It is located by first injecting a few drops of anesthetic solution into the general area. The foramen is approximately 0.5 cm anterior and in line with the hamular process, which is readily palpable as a projection immediately posterior to the end of the hard palate and medial to the alveolar process. Thus the hamular process serves as a reliable guide for this injection.

In a study by Malamed and Trieger, in 204 western skulls, the foramen was *never* found anterior to the second molar.[1] In 39% of the skulls it was located immediately adjacent to the palatal root of the second molar; in 50%, it was between the palatal roots of the second and third molars; in 10% it was found to be posterior to the palatal root of the wisdom tooth. The greater palatine foramen was *always* in line with a sagittal plane defined by the tip of the hamular process (Fig.4-2).

The greater palatine canal is short and angles backward and upward 45 degrees to the palatal

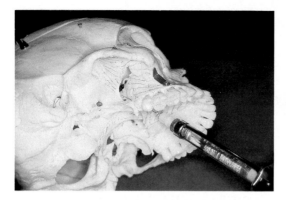

Fig. 4-1. Greater palatine foramen injection: the needle tip reaches just below the maxillary nerve trunk in the pterygomaxillary fossa.

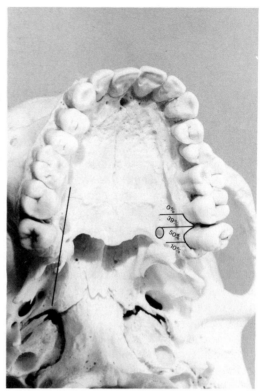

Fig. 4-2. Location of the greater palatine foramen and its relationship to the hamular process.

plane (Fig. 4-3). In this same study 97% of the canals were patent and permitted the passage of a 25-gauge needle without resistance. Jorgensen and Hayden had shown that in 15% of skulls examined, the canal leading posteriorly and superiorly from the foramen was not patent.[2] In clinical practice, when the canals are patent, the needle is advanced into the foramen 1.0 to 1.5 cm, and approximately 0.75 to 1.0 ml of anesthetic solution is injected slowly, after aspirating, to avoid intravascular injection. The anesthetic will quickly reach the sphenopalatine ganglion, which is a parasympathetic (secretomotor) extension of the facial nerve (VII). This ganglion is suspended from the maxillary nerve trunk, in the pterygomaxillary fossa. The onset of maxillary anesthesia is rapid (within 5 to 7 minutes) and extends from the lateral ala of the nose, the cheek, and upper lip to the midline and the entire unilateral bony hemimaxilla, including the hemipalate.

In performing this maxillary nerve block one other anatomic variable must be considered: how deep should the needle be inserted? The answer depends on the size of the patient's maxilla. Fortunately, a reliable guide is readily available because the course of the maxillary nerve proceeding peripherally within the substance of the maxillary bone is essentially hor-

izontal, and its exit at the infraorbital foramen approximates its height in the pterygomaxillary space. In our anatomic study of over 200 western skulls, the position of the infraorbital foramen relative to the marginal crest of alveolar bone in the region of the second premolar varied from 21 to 41 mm with an average height of 32 mm. (Fig. 4-4).

Clinically, one can readily palpate the infraorbital rim and measure its distance to the alveolar crest bone to arrive at a quick estimate of depth of needle penetration required. The standard 25-gauge "long" needle measures 1 5/8 inches or 32 mm—hardly long enough to cause overpenetration except in patients with very small maxillae. In fact, one of the shortcomings of this technique of utilizing the standard length needle is incomplete anesthesia of the central and lateral incisors in patients with large maxillae. Usually an anterior supplemental infiltra-

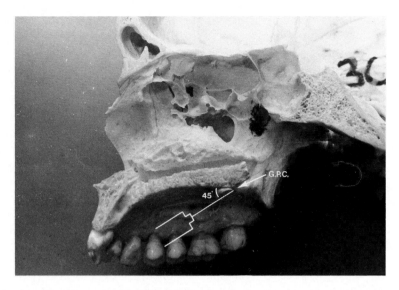

Fig. 4-3. Optimal angle of entry into greater palatine foramen.

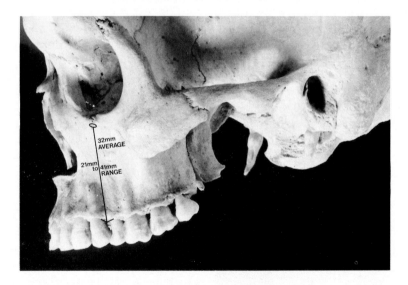

Fig. 4-4. Measurement of infraorbital foramen to maxillary alveolar crest, indicating height of the maxillary nerve anteriorly.

tion over these incisors will be required to effect complete hemimaxillary anesthesia. A second alternative is to use a longer needle in bigger patients. In general, the more peripheral nerve fibers are located closer to the center of the nerve trunk and diffusion of the anesthetic, un-less deposited close to the nerve, may never reach these deeper fibers.

Complications associated with this injection have been minor and transient. One occasion-ally sees immediate cheek blanching, indicative of inadvertent arterial perfusion. This usually fades within 4 or 5 minutes with no lasting injury. Occasionally, when overpenetration has been achieved in a small patient, transient diplopia may be experienced—resulting from some temporary paresis of extraocular muscles. This ophthalmoplegia resolves in 60 to 90 minutes. In a clinical series of over 1000 greater palatine foramen maxillary nerve blocks there were no lasting complications, infections, persistent paresthesias, or hematomas.

THE POSTERIOR TUBEROSITY INJECTION

This procedure provides the same maxillary anesthesia but approaches the pterygomaxillary fossa from the inferior lateral aspect. A 1⅝-inch (32-mm) 25-gauge disposable needle attached to an aspirating syringe is inserted approximately 1 cm lateral to the buccal sulcus. As a bony guide, the base of the zygomatic attachment to the maxilla may be used and the needle inserted posterior to this landmark. The needle is oriented superiorly and medially toward the posttuberosity area, and is advanced approximately 1¼ to 1½ inches along the periosteum. After aspiration to avoid intravascular position, 1.0 to 1.8 ml are injected slowly. Because of the medial position of the maxillary nerve trunk behind the tuberosity, a bent needle or a bent hub is advised. Disposable needles can be manually

bent to approximately 45 degrees by using a sterile gauze sponge. This will improve the access to the pterygomaxillary fossa (Fig. 4-5).

One of the disadvantages of this posterior tuberosity injection technique is the likelihood of causing a hematoma by piercing vessels in the pterygoid plexus of veins. Another disadvantage is related to the flexibility of the needle, which will often deflect posteriorly after contacting the most posterior aspect of the maxillary tuberosity. A heavier-gauge needle would be more effective (e.g., 21- or 22-gauge).

In studies of needle deflection, Jeske and Boshart showed significant deflection when using the conventional long-bevel 25- and 27-gauge needle.[3] A newer design, in which the needle end is bent toward the bevel, places the tip at approximately the center of the long axis of the needle and minimizes deflection. This newer needle is also coated with a baked-on silicone to reduce drag through tissue.

This text will repeatedly caution against intravascular injection ". . . a cartridge of procaine injected intravenously over a period of five seconds creates a rate 15 times that which is considered safe and over 200 times more toxic."[4] The amide local anesthetics used at the same concentration as procaine are even more toxic.[4] Bartlett has confirmed the work of others in showing that for nerve block anesthesia, positive aspiration is obtained in a small but significant percentage of cases.[5] This varies from 10% to 15% for mandibular blocks to 13% to 15% for maxillary and sphenopalatine nerve blocks.

Mandibular (Inferior Alveolar) Nerve Block

Blocking the inferior alveolar nerve provides anesthesia for the entire hemimandible with the exception of the lateral aspect of the mucous membrane in the molar region and cheek. This latter area requires blocking of the buccinator nerve, which is lateral to the ascending ramus of the mandible. In the performance of an inferior alveolar nerve block the lingual nerve is almost always also anesthetized. An additional infiltration injection of anesthetic is required to anesthetize the long buccal (buccinator) nerve. This is done into the soft tissues lateral and posterior to the third molar.

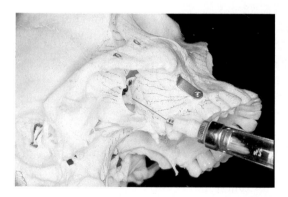

Fig. 4-5. Post-tuberosity injection: the needle is bent 45 degrees to travel along the tuberosity of the maxilla to reach the maxillary nerve trunk.

Landmarks for the inferior alveolar nerve block are readily discernible. With the patient's mouth opened widely, the operator's thumb palpates the coronoid notch along the ascending ramus of the mandible. The deepest point of this notch lines up with the bony lingula, which is immediately anterior to the nerve trunk. The operator's other fingers rest on the posterior border of the ramus and serve as a guide to the width of this bone. The foramen is usually found midway between the thumb and fingers embracing the ramus, on a line bisecting the thumbnail (Fig. 4-6).

The syringe approaches from the opposite premolar on a plane parallel to the mandibular occlusion. In this way, the prominent internal oblique ridge of bone of the ramus is avoided. When the needle has penetrated mucosa, a few drops of anesthetic solution are deposited and the needle is advanced until reaching the mid ramus. It is then withdrawn slightly and aspiration is performed. If a 25-gauge needle is used, aspiration will be more reliable and will be found to be positive, with blood coming back into the syringe in approximately 15% of inferior alveolar injections. The needle is moved slightly and again aspiration is performed. Approximately 1 ml of solution is deposited when the aspiration is negative for blood.

With the use of today's potent local anesthetics, there is no need to arbitrarily inject all of the contents of the cartridge that the manufacturer provides. If 1 ml produces adequate anesthesia, 2 ml is "overkill" and increases the hazards and toxicity potential. One can always reinject additional solution *without pain* if it becomes necessary. If the manufacturer provided cartridges of local anesthetic in 5-ml amounts instead of the standard 1.8 to 2.2 ml, it is likely that the entire contents would be used almost routinely even though a small fraction of the total dose would produce adequate anesthesia.

Classic teachings of nerve block techniques have usually stressed the importance of position of the patient. One often reads of the need to position the patient with the occlusal plane parallel to the floor. This teaching is erroneous and should be abandoned. Most modern offices use a contour-type chair with the patient tipped back into a semisupine position. Physiologically this is better than the bolt-upright position, which encourages dependent pooling of blood and promotes hypotension and syncope. Orientation for injections should be related strictly to the plane of occlusion of the teeth or other bony landmarks, regardless of the patient's head or body position, and need never relate to the floor, the ceiling, or any other outside structure.

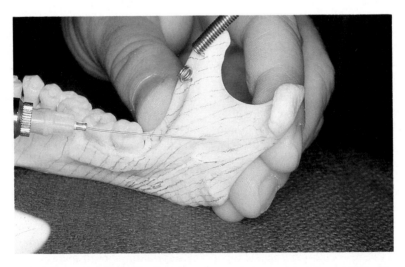

Fig. 4-6. Inferior alveolar nerve block: the fingers embrace the ramus and the needle approaches on a line from the opposite premolars, bisecting the thumbnail.

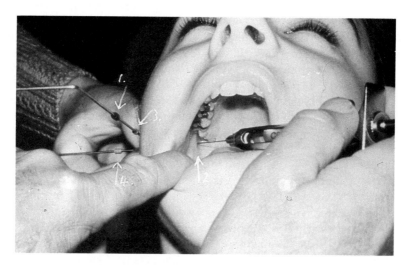

Fig. 4-7. Gow-Gates "mandibular" nerve block using intraoral and extraoral landmarks. (Courtesy Dr. George Gow-Gates.)

GOW-GATES MANDIBULAR NERVE BLOCK

From a far-off corner of our world, George A. E. Gow-Gates of Parramatta, Australia, introduced a new technique to achieve mandibular nerve anesthesia in 1973.[6] It has proved to be consistently reliable, reproducible, and associated with a better incidence of anesthesia as well as a lower incidence of complications. It has been supported by anatomic dissections by Watson[7] as well as a number of clinical studies in adults[8,9] and children.[10]

These and other studies show a consistently higher rate of successful mandibular anesthesia (96% to 98%) with the Gow-Gates block when compared to the conventional inferior alveolar block (65% to 85%). All the branches of the third division of the trigeminal nerve (V) that traverse the pterygomandibular space are anesthetized, including the lingual and buccinator as well as the inferior alveolar branches. Occasionally, the buccinator nerve will require a supplementary infiltration of local anesthetic proximal and lateral to the third molar. Onset of anesthesia is relatively rapid, usually within 2 to 3 minutes, and often is experienced as a progression from proximal to peripheral areas (centrifugal). When complete (5 to 7 minutes) pulpal anesthesia of the ipsilateral incisors is confirmed, without evidence of crossover of the midline.

The technique is not difficult and depends on extraoral and intraoral landmarks. The ultimate aim is to deposit the anesthetic solution precisely at the condylar neck, where there is a distinct bony endpoint, usually at a needle depth of 25 to 27 mm.

GOW-GATES TECHNIQUE

With the patient's mouth held wide open, the medial side of the deep tendon of the temporalis muscle is identified. The syringe is placed at the opposite corner of the mouth, over the opposite canine and premolar teeth, and the needle penetrates tissue medial to the temporalis tendon and just below the occlusal plane of the maxillary second molar. The path of the needle is directed toward the tragal notch of the ear on a line connecting the corner of the mouth with the tragus. The patient or the operator may insert a finger in the external auditory meatus to serve as a more visible guide. The needle is advanced along this plane until bone is contacted. Failure to contact bone at 25 to 27 mm indicates the need to redirect the needle rather than to deposit solution through the sigmoid notch and into the masseter muscle (Fig. 4-7).

Aspiration should always precede injection. Occasionally, a positive aspiration may indicate penetration of the internal maxillary artery, which is passing from lateral to medial at the level of the condylar neck. With the mouth opened wide, the condyle moves forward and away from the artery. Usually, 1.8 to 2.2 ml has been found to provide adequate to profound anesthesia in over 96% of cases.

MANDIBULAR ANESTHESIA: AKINOSI-VASIRANI TECHNIQUE

This technique has been particularly recommended when the patient presents with limited mandibular opening. The syringe is held parallel to the occlusal plane and the needle penetrates tissue at the level of the mucogingival junction of the maxillary third molar, just medial to the mandibular ramus.[11] It is advanced approximately 1½ inch. After aspiration the anesthetic solution is deposited. The needle tip should be in the pterygomandibular space just superior to the lingula. Onset of tongue anesthesia is rapid, with mandibular anesthesia following within 4 to 5 minutes. In a limited clinical series[12] there was no evidence of untoward complications such as trismus, hematoma, postinjection infection, etc. The authors suggest that the deposition of anesthetic solution with Akinosi technique approximates that achieved by the Gow-Gates method and results in an equivalent level of good anesthesia.

Infraorbital Nerve Block

This regional nerve block anesthetizes the anterior and middle superior alveolar nerves of the maxilla in addition to the inferior palpebral, lateral nasal, and superior labial nerves. It is usually sufficient for operative dentistry on the unilateral incisors, canines, and premolars. It does not provide the palatal anesthesia necessary for surgical treatment. Additional infiltration into the palate is required to block this area completely.

The technique involves identifying the infraorbital foramen by palpation. It is usually found approximately 0.5 to 1.0 cm inferior to the infraorbital notch and rim, in line with the second premolar. A 25-gauge 1⅝-inch disposable needle attached to an aspirating syringe is inserted over the second premolar 0.5 cm lateral to the alveolar bone. It is slowly advanced and a few drops of anesthetic expressed. The needle tip comes to rest under the palpating

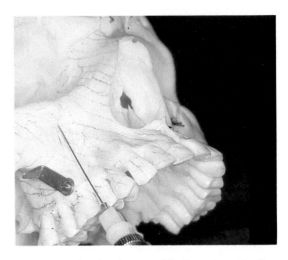

Fig. 4-8. Infraorbital nerve block: syringe in line with second premolar with needle tip approximately 1 cm below orbital rim.

finger that has identified the infraorbital foramen. A small amount of solution is injected. The needle is then advanced again into the foramen with the fingertip held firmly to facilitate the solution going into the anterior portion of the infraorbital canal (Fig. 4-8). After aspiration, 0.5 to 0.75 ml of anesthetic is injected. The roof of the infraorbital canal will limit intrusion of the needle and prevent damage to the globe of the eye. The syringe barrel is in contact with the lower lip and angled slightly anteriorly because the foramen opening is oriented more toward the midline. Jorgensen suggests that for children this one injection will provide anesthesia to all primary teeth in that hemimaxilla.[2]

Nasopalatine Nerve Block

This block anesthetizes the nasopalatine nerve, which supplies the anterior hard palate. It is a painful injection and methods to diminish the discomfort include applying a topical anesthetic, using a jet injection, or preliminarily infiltrating a minute amount of solution into the overlying mucosa. This technique involves inserting the needle into the papilla *parallel* to the labial alveolar plate of bone. It is advanced into the incisive canal for about 1 cm, and 0.25 to 0.5 ml of solution is slowly injected after aspiration (Fig. 4-9).

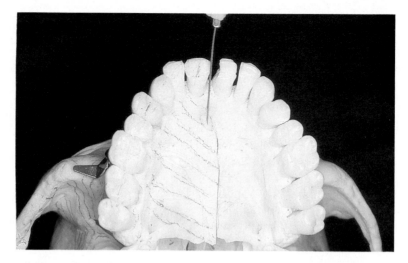

Fig. 4-9. Nasopalatine nerve block: needle in line with labial alveolar plate of bone.

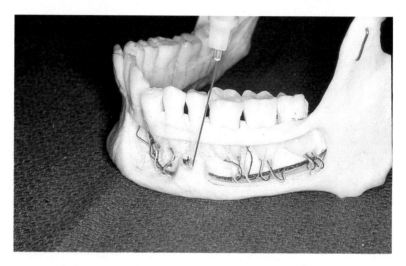

Fig. 4-10. Mental nerve injection: needle aligned with second premolar.

Mental Nerve Block

The mental nerve exits from the mandibular canal at the mental foramen, in the region of the mandibular first and second premolars, to innervate the lower lip and mucosa anterior to the foramen. The needle is inserted into the area of the apex of the second premolar. Because the opening of the canal is usually oriented posteriorly, the syringe should be directed from a position slightly distal and lateral to the second premolar (Fig. 4-10). A small amount of anesthetic solution, 0.5 ml, will suffice.

Infiltration Anesthesia

Paraperiosteal injections over the apices of individual teeth are routinely used for conservative dentistry, especially in the maxilla. They usually provide adequate local analgesia and obviate the need for block anesthesia. The amount of solution required is small; usually 0.5 ml or less is adequate. Injecting more anesthetic can be done secondarily if prolonged treatment is needed or the level of analgesia is inadequate. This approach is preferable to using more drug than necessary at the time of the ini-

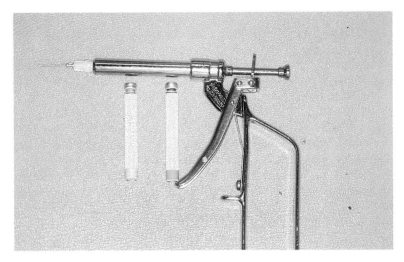

Fig. 4-11. Hydraulic pressure syringe is a helpful adjunct to delivering the small amount of anesthetic required for single-tooth anesthesia.

tial injection. Reinjection is usually pain free.

In the mandible, infiltration anesthesia is often inadequate for good analgesia, and multiple injections, including pericemental injections, are less desirable than one highly effective inferior alveolar nerve block. The duration of analgesia may vary depending upon the agent used and the epinephrine content of the solution. Duration of action will be discussed further in following sections.

Pericemental or Intraligamentary Injections

With the introduction of hydraulic, high-pressure syringes, it has become easier to obtain regionally limited local anesthesia to obtund pain.[13] In effect, these injections, initiated into the periodontal ligament space, are really intrabony injections and do not stay confined to the tooth. A reasonably high rate of successful and brief anesthesia (65% to 80%) for 15 to 30 minutes permits single-tooth anesthesia for a variety of procedures. Several favorable features exist. A minute amount of anesthetic solution (0.2 to 0.4 ml) will often suffice; generalized and prolonged numbness of adjacent tissues is avoided; no permanent injury is caused to either pulp[14] or the periodontal ligament.[15] A recent extension of this technique by Saadoun

and Malamed[16] has been the intraseptal-intrabony injection for periodontal surgery. The point of puncture, with a short 27-gauge needle, is through the interdental papilla, into the interproximal alveolar bone, and into the bony marrow space. Resistance to the flow of the anesthetic solution is a requisite to effective anesthesia in both the intraligamental and intraseptal injections. The onset of anesthesia is usually immediate, with a success rate of 92% with the first injection. The author has frequently used intraligamentary injections as a supplement to incomplete nerve block anesthesia, with marked success; especially in cases where a "hot tooth" requiring nerve extirpation or extraction warranted deeper analgesia (Fig. 4-11).

Local Anesthetic Solutions

Although many local anesthetics have been synthesized, only a few have been accepted for widespread clinical use. Their rate of success in obtunding pain is remarkably high, and often their effectiveness is further enhanced by adjunctive aids such as nitrous oxide–oxygen psychosedation and intravenous sedation. Whereas the local anesthetic serves to block painful stimuli, the emotional reaction to dental treatment is ameliorated by these adjuncts, making the local anesthetic more effective.

Local anesthetics are of three chemical types: ester type compounds (e.g., procaine); amide type compounds (e.g., lidocaine); and hydroxy compounds (e.g., benzocaine). The latter are used primarily for topical analgesia. Injectable local anesthetics are weakly basic and poorly soluble in water. They are used as hydrochloride salts, which are acidic and more water soluble. In general, the potency of an anesthetic parallels its toxicity. Tissue compatibility of commonly used local anesthetics is good, although degenerative changes occur at the local site of injection,[17,18] particularly within muscle, and evidence of microscarring is found. Epinephrine and other agents producing vasoconstriction significantly augmented lidocaine myotoxicity.[19] Toxicity is usually related to intravascular injection, which compromises both the cardiovascular and central nervous systems.[20]

Lipid solubility of these anesthetic compounds is the most important determinant of potency. In the ester series, tetracaine hydrochloride is more lipid soluble and more potent than procaine hydrochloride. In the amide series, bupivacaine hydrochloride is 35 times more lipid soluble than mepivacaine hydrochloride and four times more potent. Etidocaine hydrochloride is 50 times more lipid soluble and four times more potent than lidocaine hydrochloride.[21] The duration of effectiveness of the anesthetic agent is largely determined by the extent of its protein binding, in the lipo-protein membrane of the nerve cell. Tetracaine, which is 10 times more highly bound to protein, has a duration of action that is three to four times that of procaine. Bupivacaine and etidocaine, in the amide group, are over 90% bound to protein as compared to their analogues, mepivacaine and lidocaine, which are 65% to 75% protein bound. The former provide two to three times the anesthetic duration when compared to mepivacaine and lidocaine.

Clinically, these agents may be categorized into three groups according to potency and duration: (1) low potency and short duration, as represented by procaine and chloroprocaine

hydrochloride; (2) intermediate potency and duration as represented by lidocaine, mepivacaine, and prilocaine hydrochloride; and (3) high potency and long duration, represented by tetracaine, bupivacaine, and etidocaine. Onset of action varies with each agent—shortest for chloroprocaine and longest for tetracaine.[21]

The addition of a vasoconstrictor to the local anesthetic solution serves to enhance the duration of action by retarding or decreasing vascular absorption, making more drug available for nerve uptake and conduction blockade. In general, infiltration anesthesia without vasoconstrictor added to those amides with intermediate potency and duration (lidocaine and mepivacaine) lasts 20 to 60 minutes, whereas conduction block lasts 45 to 180 minutes. There is considerable individual variation of effect and duration shown by all local anesthetic agents.

The presence of a vasoconstrictor also effectively limits the amount of anesthetic absorbed into the general circulation in a given time and lessens the possibility of systemic toxicity. With an extravascular injection, the amount of vasoconstrictor entering the blood circulation is estimated to be 1 µg/min. This represents less than 10% of the endogenous epinephrine or norepinephrine produced according to Glover.[22] Apprehension and poor anesthesia may provoke far more epinephrine release than can be absorbed from an extravascularly deposited solution of local anesthetic with a vasoconstrictor, although modest increases are noted in stroke volume and cardiac output.

The addition of epinephrine 1:100,000 per ml prolongs the action of infiltrated lidocaine from 30 minutes to approximately 150 minutes. Increasing the concentration of epinephrine to 1:50,000 per ml hastens the onset of analgesia and further prolongs the duration of action. Other vasoconstrictors such as Levophed, Neo-Cobefrin, and Neo-Synephrine are used with local anesthetics to decrease the likelihood of rapid absorption that may precipitate systematic reactions as well as prolong the local anesthetic effect.

Depending on the site of injection, the peak blood level of the anesthetic will be 0.5 to 2.0 µg/ml for each 100 mg of lidocaine hydrochloride or mepivacaine hydrochloride. For most healthy adults, evidence of toxicity begins to appear at blood levels approximating 5 μg/ml. Early clinical manifestations include dizziness; paresthesias of face, lips, and fingers; tinnitus; disorientation; and cardiac dysrhythmia—progressing to unconsciousness, respiratory depression, tremors, convulsions, and coma. Early signs of central nervous system excitation are caused by initial selective blockade of inhibitory neurons, allowing facilitory fibers to function unopposed. With increasing blood and brain levels, depression supervenes with blockade of facilitory neurons as well. In the presence of diazepam, the threshold for lidocaine toxicity is elevated. Vasoconstrictors serve to delay the uptake and thereby significantly reduce the peak blood level of local anesthetics deposited extravascularly.

In a survey of adverse reactions to local anesthetic/vasoconstrictor preparations, Boakes et al found that the factor common to these recorded adverse reactions was the high concentration of vasoconstrictors.[23] Safety considerations dictate that concentrations of epinephrine not exceed 1:100,000 and that the use of 1:50,000 be reserved for special problems. This is consonant with the pharmacotherapeutic maxim to use the smallest quantity and lowest concentration of the least toxic anesthetic that will accomplish the job. Brown has shown that there is a lack of significant clinical difference between lidocaine hydrochloride test solutions containing epinephrine in 12.5, 10.0, and 5.0 μg/ml amounts.[24] There was, however a greater, incidence of the "alarm syndrome" in patients receiving the higher epinephrine concentrations. Gross et al showed that an intravenous bolus of lidocaine hydrochloride 1.5 mg/kg given to healthy unpremedicated volunteers caused a transient respiratory depression and did not change heart rate, blood pressure, or state of consciousness.[25] They caution of the possible potentiation of this depressant effect when superimposed on sedated or anesthetized patients.

It has been proposed that one route of high anesthetic brain level may be caused by inadvertent vascular injection into the external ca-

rotid artery, which, in retrograde fashion, would enter the internal carotid artery.[26] This "reverse carotid flow theory" was challenged by Yagiella, who showed that bolus injections given intravenously proved to be more toxic (in rats) than when given directly to the brain via the internal carotid artery injection.[27] The coadministration of epinephrine increased the lethality of intravascular lidocaine by 50% to 60%.

In this regard, it is important to cite the potential harm of large amounts of epinephrine delivered to the bloodstream by their presence in the local anesthetic or when applied topically to the mucous membranes. Hilley et al reported a fatality associated with the use of epinephrine-impregnated gingival retraction cord used in crown-and-bridge procedures.[28] Many patients report "palpitations" when this 8% racemic epinephrine cord is used, reflecting a rapid uptake of this systemically acting adrenergic stimulant.

Mulroy and Halcomb have recently shown that the addition of 1:200,000 epinephrine to lidocaine provided optimal vasoconstriction in cutaneous capillary blood flow when compared to 1:50,000 and 1:100,000 concentrations, within a 2-hour time frame.[29] They concluded that "there is no apparent justification for greater than 1:200,000 epinephrine concentration in subcutaneous infiltration."

Tolas, Pflug, and Halter studied the plasma epinephrine concentration in healthy clinical subjects receiving lidocaine with and without epinephrine (1:100,000).[30] Only those patients receiving the combination injection (epinephrine, 18 μg) showed a significant increase in epinephrine level when compared to preinjection baseline and to nonepinephrine controls.

After 5 minutes, the systemic blood pressure in patients receiving the lidocaine-epinephrine combination was significantly lower than the controls. The potential for adverse cardiodynamic effects was suggested in medically compromised patients receiving greater amounts of lidocaine with epinephrine.

Allen[31] showed that with the use of only 1.8 ml of 2% lidocaine hydrochloride with 1:100,000 epinephrine, there is a rise of 18% to 24% in stroke volume of the heart, reflecting the beta-adrenergic effect of this small amount of epinephrine in a patient under general anesthesia.

Mechanism of Action

Local anesthetics are believed to reversibly affect the permeability of the plasma membrane surrounding the nerve. This decrease in permeability to sodium and potassium is achieved by altering calcium at its binding sites in the lipoprotein layer. The cation released by the local anesthetic salt binds to the receptor sites, displacing calcium.

In 1963, Drs. Eccles, Hodgkins, and Huxley were awarded the Nobel Prize for their work on the ionic mechanisms involved in nerve conduction and inhibition. They demonstrated that nerve cell bodies contained numerous small knoblike endings on the terminal branches of their axons, the sites for synapses. A 70-angstrom capsule surrounds these small synaptic knobs, which contain numerous vesicles believed to be packages of specific chemicals for nerve transmission. This surface membrane separates two aqueous solutions of very different ionic composition. The interior solution has a high concentration of potassium and low sodium. The exterior solution is opposite in electrolyte concentrations. Depolarization of the membrane is accompanied by a change in these concentrations.[32] Molecules closely related chemically and sterically to acetylcholine block electrical activity along the axon as well as at the synaptic junction. These findings support the concept that acetylcholine mediates axonal conduction.

Sax and Pletcher had proposed that local anesthetics inhibit nerve conduction by replacing calcium ions in the formation of a more stable complex with phospholipids in the neural membrane.[33] They suggest that the local anesthetic acts as a hydrogen bond donor and forms this complex with a receptor in the membrane. The assumption is that such a complex inhibits and competes with acetylcholine to block transmission. Different types of fibers in a mixed nerve are affected to varying degrees. Motor function usually remains intact for some time after all sensation is lost. In general, large fibers are more resistant to inhibitory drug effects whereas efferent fibers are more resistant than afferent fibers and myelinated more resistant than nonmyelinated. Recently, Gissen, Covino, and Gregus have shown that the larger, faster-conducting, A fibers are inhibited at a lower concentration of anesthetic than smaller fibers, contrary to prevailing thought.[34] To explain this apparent discrepancy, they suggest that smaller-diameter fibers are closer to the surface of the nerve and therefore more readily affected by the local anesthetic diffusion.

Newer studies suggest that local anesthetics may work by interfering with the conversion of the sol-to-gel phase of the membrane lipid and thus alter the conformational changes in protein necessary for opening the sodium channels. Others indicate that the neutral and ionized forms of local anesthetics may have different binding sites on the channel or separate receptor sites.[35]

The lung has been found to play an active role in the binding of local anesthetics introduced into the bloodstream. More than 90% of intravascular lidocaine was taken up by lung tissue and then released into the bloodstream over the next 30 seconds, thus decreasing the initial peak level. Another mechanism that serves to "tie up" local anesthetic compounds in the blood and tissues is their protein binding, especially to alpha,-acid glycoprotein. Protein binding may be significantly depressed in situations of anesthetic overdosage and acidosis.[35]

Selected Agents

The development of newer local anesthetic agent and techniques of administration has significantly expanded the success rate and flexibility of local anesthetic usage. Agents are now readily available to achieve 20 to 30 minutes of profound anesthesia to up to 8 to 12 hours of postsurgical relief of pain.

Lidocaine (Xylocaine), the first nonester-type local anesthetic introduced into clinical practice, withstands boiling and autoclaving. It diffuses rapidly and gives a rapid onset of action. The suggested maximum dosage is approximately 300 to 400 mg (15 ml to 20 ml of a 2% solution).

Mepivacaine (Carbocaine) is also a nonester compound that can be boiled or autoclaved. Its action is very similar to that of lidocaine. It is used in a 3% concentration without vasoconstrictor or 2% with 1:20,000 levonordefrin (Neo-Cobefrin), which provides a longer duration of action. Prilocaine (Citanest) is an amide that is often used in 4% concentration without a vasoconstrictor to produce up to 60 to 90 minutes of infiltration anesthesia. The potency of prilocaine is said to be only 0.6 that of lidocaine, but it is cleared less rapidly from the injection site, probably related in part to the fact that its vasodilator effect is only half that of lidocaine. By the addition of a small amount of adrenaline (1:200,000 per ml) its action is lengthened by 20 to 30 minutes.[36, 37] The suggested maximum dosage of a 4% solution is 400 mg or 10 ml. Studies have indicated that serum levels of prilocaine decrease much more rapidly than lidocaine. A few instances of cyanosis have been recorded in man when the maximum dose of 400 mg was exceeded. This was attributed to the formation of methemoglobin from a derivative of prilocaine. In the usual small clinical doses used in dentistry, this should not occur because this adverse effect is dose related.

Bupivacaine (Marcaine), a highly lipid-soluble, potent, long-acting local anesthetic, belongs to the amide series. It is an analogue of mepivacaine. It is presently available as a 0.5% solution (5 mg/ml) plain and with 1:200,000 epinephrine. It has been shown to be highly effective in providing analgesia for surgical procedures and for a protracted pain-free postoperative period following block injection. Trieger and Gillen showed a significant decrease in the number of postoperative doses of analgesics required when bupivacaine anesthesia was compared to mepivacaine.[38] Mean onset time to achieve surgical block anesthesia was approximately 2 minutes longer than for mepivacaine. Duration of anesthesia was twice that of mepivacaine for plain bupivacaine and almost two and one half times longer when 1:200,000 epinephrine was added to the bupivacaine.

As with all local anesthetics, there was considerable individual variation ranging from 4 to 11 hours of anesthesia. These data and subsequent studies suggested that even longer durations were achieved by increasing the total dose

of bupivacaine administered. Giving 15 to 20 mg of bupivacaine hydrochloride with 1:200,000 epinephrine consistently provided 8 to 12 hours of conduction anesthesia and pain relief. Unlike lidocaine or mepivacaine, duration of anesthesia appears to be distinctly affected by the dosage deposited, probably because of its high lipid solubility and high protein binding. It has also been suggested that a period of analgesia may extend beyond the point of return of normal sensation.[39] Maximum single doses of bupivacaine hydrochloride for the average adult should not exceed 100 mg.

Concern has been raised in anesthesiology circles about the cardiotoxicity of larger doses of bupivacaine. Clarkson and Hondeghem have shown that bupivacaine causes cardiac conduction depression by blocking the sodium channel in what is called a "fast in–slow out" fashion, whereas lidocaine blocks the channel in a "fast in–fast out" manner.[40] They caution against high circulating blood levels of bupivacaine, which may produce depression for longer periods and be difficult to reverse. In dentistry, doses are usually well below these toxic levels, especially if care is exercised to aspirate and avoid intravascular injections.

Etidocaine (Duranest), a highly lipid-soluble, potent analogue of lidocaine, has been compared to bupivacaine. There are some subtle differences in rate of onset and duration of anesthesia. In a double-blind study by Davis, Oakley, and Smith for oral surgery, two solutions were compared: lidocaine hydrochloride 2% (20 mg/ml) with 1:100,000 epinephrine and etidocaine 1.5% (15 mg/ml), with 1:200,000 epinephrine.[41] Lip numbness on the etidocaine-injected side lasted twice as long as the lidocaine-treated side and the pain-free postoperative period was also twice as long.

With infiltration anesthesia, Danielsson, Evers, and Nordenram compared bupivacaine, etidocaine, and lidocaine.[42] A longer duration of pain-free postoperative time with bupivacaine was found. Interestingly, lidocaine provided the longest duration of *pulpal* anesthesia compared to the two other long-acting agents. They hypothesized that the lipid solubility of both etidocaine and bupivacaine may decrease its diffusion and penetration to the apical area in maxillary infiltration injections when compared to lidocaine.

Related Considerations

CARPULE CONTAMINATION

Shannon and Feller have shown that storage of local anesthetic Carpules in alcohol, which is a common practice, may be a source of contamination.[43] Over a period of time the alcohol slowly enters the Carpule through the rubber stopper end. If this continues for a long time a deleterious amount of alcohol may be injected along with the anesthetic solution. It is suggested that either the Carpules be stored with only the needle-contacting end in preservative solution or, better still, that each sterile Carpule be placed in a sterile envelope to be dispensed as needed.

It must be emphasized that each sterile cartridge of local anesthetic solution is intended for only one patient and never to be "saved" and administered to another patient. Cross-contamination and possible infection dictate the simple prudent policy of discarding each unexpended cartridge. Similarly, each disposable needle used may be used repeatedly, but only for the same patient, at that visit. It is false economy and unethical to risk reuse of a nonresterilizable needle.

ALLERGIC REACTIONS

Methylparaben used in minute amounts in anesthetic solutions as a preservative has been implicated in a few cases of allergic reactions that had been attributed erroneously to the primary anesthetic ingredient. This preservative is chemically related to para-aminobenzoic acid, and to procaine.[44]

There are unfortunately many patients who are told that they are "allergic" to the local anesthetic when, in fact, they may have experienced a syncopal episode or even an intravascular injection with the probability of near-toxic overdose. While fainting and syncope are not uncommon in the dental office, their incidence has markedly decreased with the introduction of the contour chair, which provides for elevation of the legs and avoids dependent blood pooling with subsequent hypotension, cerebral ischemia, syncope, and even convulsions. Currently, none of the amide local anesthetics used in dental cartridges contain methylparaben.

True allergy to an amide-type local anesthetic is so rare as to be considered reportable. There are a few approaches to be taken for the patient allegedly allergic to local anesthesia. A precise history of the event is necessary, as is communicating with the practitioner to determine which specific agent(s) were used and the reactions observed. One method that has been used with limited effect but may avoid the need for general anesthesia whenever dental work is required is to find another drug with local anesthetic properties.

Diphenhydramine hydrochloride (Benadryl) is an antihistamine drug that has been recommended for its local anesthetic properties, particularly for use in patients suspected of being allergic to the usual local anesthetics. A 1% solution has greater tissue-irritating qualities when compared to 2% procaine although it is more potent. Using a 1% solution of diphenhydramine hydrochloride with 1:100,000 epinephrine, Malamed obtained profound dental anesthesia, within 5 minutes, which lasted 30 to 40 minutes.[45] This agent provoked a burning sensation on injection into a number of patients receiving a mandibular nerve block.

Skin and mucosal testings of the presumed allergen(s) has not been entirely reliable. Usually the most effective way to rule out the presumed hypersensitivity is to challenge the patient with the agent—but with all necessary safeguards and personnel available should an acute anaphylactoid reaction precipitate. This may be done in an anesthesia treatment or induction room or recovery room.

In my consultation practice, I have evaluated 31 patients referred because of local anesthetic "allergy" or "bad reaction." After reviewing of the history the patient is placed in a dental chair, tipped backwards, and vital signs are taken. An intravenous line is established with a venipuncture and a saline drip is started. The patient is then given a small amount of diazepam or midazolam to effect a light sedation. Next, a syringe of 1:1,000 epinephrine is drawn up and set aside. A vial of cardiac lidocaine (lidocaine hydrochloride 2%) without preservatives, or epinephrine, is drawn into a small disposable syringe and approximately 0.5 ml is injected over the maxillary canine area. Vital signs are repeated. Oxygen and cardiopulmonary equipment are available, but they have never been needed for these 31 individuals, who were found not to be allergic to lidocaine.

There are several categories of people who fall into this group. Most of them are extremely apprehensive. Some are truly hyperreactors with a hypersensitive carotid sinus reflex that throws them into bradycardia and hypotension. These patients should be given atropine or glycopyrolate, to block the overactive vagus nerve and reflex, and horizontally positioned before being injected. A very few patients release histamine under stress and show idiopathic angioedema, which can be minimized with oral or intravenous diphenhydramine or other antihistamine.

NEEDLE BREAKAGE

The incidence of breakage of hypodermic needles during the administration of local anesthesia has significantly decreased since the introduction of disposable needles. Nevertheless, the rare case report recalls the caution that must be exercised, especially when treating children.[46] Needles should be of sufficient length so that they are never inserted to the hub to achieve the required depth of penetration. The operator must anticipate unexpected movements by the child and may consider preoperative sedation as an adjunct to local anesthesia.

Menske and Gowgiel point out that the depth of needle penetration for performing an inferior alveolar nerve block is usually equal to half the distance across the mandibular ramus (anteroposteriorly), with an average of 16 mm.[47] Short needles deflect less than longer ones and still afford adequate exposure of the nonburied portion. They also note that disposable needles, unlike older ones, incorporate the hub and extend through it into the anesthetic cartridge, thus reinforcing this potentially fragile area.

In a clinical study comparing 25-, 27-, and 30-gauge needles, it was determined that the six participating, blindfolded dentists were "never aware of which needle was used" when injected in the retromolar area to a depth of 2 to 3 mm.[48]

HEMOPHILIC PATIENTS

Special consideration must be given to the use of local anesthesia in hemophilic patients. Mandibular nerve block anesthesia is avoided unless the patient is receiving factor VIII (antihemophilic globulin) to raise his titer.[49] Serious sequelae involving large hematomas that encroach on the airway have been reported in improperly prepared hemophilic patients. Fig. 4-12 shows ecchymoses resulting from an infiltration anesthetic given for conservative dentistry; although this was not life-threatening it represented a mild complication. Alternative methods to local anesthesia should be sought in

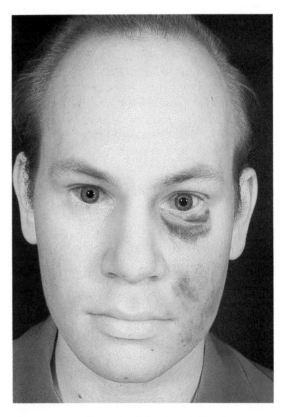

Fig. 4-12. Ecchymosis following infiltration anesthesia in a hemophilic boy.

the treatment of hemophilic patients. Nitrous oxide–oxygen sedation is often well tolerated and may obviate the need for local anesthetic injections when conservative dental treatment is performed. General anesthesia (without nasal intubation) is recommended for dental surgical management of the hemophilic patient, together with supplemental factor VIII administration and epsilon-aminocaproic acid (EACA) to prevent fibrinolysis of the clot.[50]

OTHER COMPLICATIONS

Complications of local anesthetic administration are infrequent. Some patients experience a protracted period of paresthesia if the nerve trunk has been traumatized during injections. Of course, the contamination of the contents of the anesthetic Carpule with alcohol from the storage solution may also be a cause of neural damage and paresthesia.[43] A hematoma may result from trauma to regional blood vessels. The use of aspirating syringes should decrease this complication. Local pressure and ice packs to the area of swelling are recommended to limit the extent of the selling. Subsequently, hot packs are used to aid in the resolution of the hematoma and to encourage normal muscle function.

Occasionally trismus follows inferior alveolar nerve block injections, which usually subsides within 24 to 48 hours. Rarely such a complication will become more marked as the trismus intensifies. In the absence of sepsis (no fever, pain, erythema, lymphadenopathy), oral physiotherapy to encourage gradual and progressive mouth opening is important. This may be done with the use of multiple tongue blades wedged between the teeth, or a rubber stopper device to encourage the patient to practice stretching exercises. In addition, the use of hot packs to the jaw and the administration of an anti-inflammatory, analgesic agent are helpful. If little progress in mouth opening is achieved, the patient may require forced opening under a general anesthetic with subsequent vigorous muscle physiotherapy. If allowed to persist, the original hematoma organizes and then becomes fibrotic with greater limitation of function a lasting likelihood.

Sepsis resulting from a contaminated needle also leads to a difficult, deep-seated infection of the pterygomandibular space. This condition is rare and may require aggressive antibiotic treatment as well as surgical drainage of the appropriate fascial spaces. Faulty technique associated with inferior alveolar nerve block may lead to anesthesia of the motor branches of the facial nerve (VII). This can occur if the needle is advanced too far, reaching posterior to the mandibular ramus. The patient may develop a transient inability to close the eyelid. Diplopia may also result from anesthetization of branches of the extrinsic muscles of the eye.

Occasionally, when a maxillary tuberosity injection is being administered, the patient reports instantaneous burning in the area of distribution of the infraorbital nerve, and the skin of the cheek blanches. The rapidity of response and the vasoconstriction of the skin vessels indicates an intra-arterial injection which, fortunately, fades within 10 to 15 minutes without lasting sequelae.

Although anomalies of nerve and blood vessel distributions exist, the high rate of successful and safe administration of local anesthetics is well established. These facts, coupled with careful preoperative patient evaluation and preparedness for potential complications, will ensure the continued widespread use of local anesthesia in dentistry.

An interesting study by Peterson and Klein showed that warming of the anesthetic solution to body temperature (37° C) prior to injection did not influence the pain experienced and reported by their subjects, nor did it hasten the onset of anesthesia.[51]

In the future we may look forward to the availability of still other local anesthetics. Articane hydrochloride (Ultracaine) is an amide with very rapid onset of action and is highly diffusible through soft tissue and bone. It may provide palatal anesthesia when injected into the maxillary buccal area. Methemoglobinemia may occur with high doses of the drug. Dental cartridges are available in Europe and Canada but not yet in the United States.[52,53]

Summary

Local anesthesia has had a profound influence on the acceptance and practice of dentistry in the past 70 years. New and standard techniques of injection are described for the control of pain mediated by fibers of the trigeminal (V) nerve. Maxillary and mandibular nerve blocks, rather than multiple injections, are advocated to achieve the same anesthetic coverage when extensive work is planned. The routine use of an aspirating syringe is advocated for all local anesthetic administrations to prevent intravascular injection and toxic overdose of drug. Current hypotheses of local anesthetic action are presented. A few selected agents are discussed as well as special considerations related to their use.

References

1. Malamed SF, Trieger, N: Intraoral maxillary nerve block: an anatomical and clinical study, *Anesth Prog* 30:2, 44-48, 1983.

2. Jorgensen NB, Hayden J: *Sedation, local and general anesthesia in dentistry,* ed 3, Philadelphia, 1980, Lea & Febiger.

3. Jeske AH, Boshart BF: Deflection of conventional versus nonconventional dental needles in vitro, *Anesth Prog* 32:2, 62-64, 1985.

4. American Dental Association: *Accepted dental therapeutics,* ed 34, Chicago, 1971-1972, American Dental Association.

5. Bartlett SZ: Clinical observations on the effects of injections of local anesthetic preceded by aspiration, *Oral Surg Oral Med Oral Pathol* 33:520-526, 1972.

6. Gow-Gates GAE: Mandibular conduction anesthesia: a new technique using extraoral landmarks, *Oral Surg Oral Med Oral Pathol* 36:3, 321-328, 1973.

7. Watson JE: Appendix: Some anatomic aspects of the Gow-Gates technique for mandibular anesthesia, *Oral Surg Oral Med Oral Pathol* 36:3, 328-330, 1973.

8. Malamed SF: The Gow-Gates mandibular block: evaluation after 4,275 cases, *Oral Surg Oral Med Oral Pathol* 51:5, 463-467, 1981.

9. Levy TP: An assessment of the Gow-Gates mandibular block for third molar surgery, *J Am Dent Assoc* 103:37-39, 1981.

10. Yamada A, Jastak JT: Clinical evaluation of the Gow-Gates block in children, *Anesth Prog* 28(4):106-109, 1981.

11. Akinosi JO: A new approach to the mandibular nerve block, *Br J Oral Surg* 15:83-87, 1977.

12. Gustainis JF, Peterson LJ: An alternative method of mandibular nerve block, *J Am Dent Assoc* 103:33-36, 1981.

13. Malamed SF: The periodontal ligament injection: an alternative to inferior alveolar nerve block, *Oral Surg Oral Med Oral Pathol* 53(2):117-121, 1982.

14. Peurach JC: Pulpal response to intraligamentary injection in the Cynomologus monkey, *Anesth Prog* 32(2):73-75, 1985.

15. Walton RE, Garnick JJ: The periodontal ligament injection: histologic effects on the periodontium in monkeys, *J Endod* 8:22-26, 1982.

16. Saadoun AP, Malamed S: Intraseptal anesthesia in periodontal surgery, *J Am Dent Assoc* 11:249-256, 1985.

17. Dolivick MF et al: Degenerative changes in masseter muscle following injection of lidocaine: a histochemical study, *J Dent Res* 56(11):1395-1402, 1977.

18. Benoit PW: Microscarring in skeletal muscle after repeated exposures to lidocaine with epinephrine, *J Oral Surg* 36:530-533, 1978.

19. Yagiella JA, Benoit PW, Fort NF: Mechanism of epinephrine enhancement of lidocaine-induced skeletal muscle necrosis, *J Dent Res* 61(5): 686-690, 1982.

20. Adriani J, Zepernick R, Hyde E: Influence of the status of the patient on systemic effects of local anesthetic agents, *Anesth Analg* 45:87-91, 1966.

21. Covino BG, Giddon DB: Pharmacology of local anesthetic agents, *J Dent Res* 60(8):1454-1459, 1981.

22. Glover J: Vasoconstrictor in dental anesthetic contraindication—fact or fallacy? *Aust Dent J* 13 (1):65-69, 1968.

23. Boakes AJ et al: Adverse reactions to local anesthetics/vasoconstrictor preparations, *Br Dent J* 133:137-140, 1972.

24. Brown G: Lidocaine-epinephrine anesthetics for dentistry, *J Dent Res* 52(3):565-566, 1973.

25. Gross JB et al: The effect of lidocaine on the ventilatory response to carbon dioxide, *Anesthesiology* 59:521-525, 1983.

26. Aldrete JA et al: Reverse carotid flow—a possible explanation for some reactions to local anesthetics, *J Am Dent Assoc* 94:1142-1145, 1977.

27. Yagiella JA: Intravascular lidocaine toxicity: influence of epinephrine and route of administration, *Anesth Prog* 32(2):57-61, 1985.

28. Hilley MD et al: Fatality associated with the combined use of halothane and gingival retraction cord. *Anesthesiology* 60:587-588, 1984.

29. Mulroy MF, Halcomb JL: 1:200,000 epinephrine provides optimal cutaneous vasoconstriction, *Anesthesiology* 61(3):A 194, 1984.

30. Tolas AG, Pflug AE, Halter JB: Arterial plasma epinephrine concentrations and hemodynamic responses after dental injection of local anesthetic with epinephrine, *J Am Dent Assoc* 104:41-43, 1982.

31. Allen GD: Minor anesthesia, *J Oral Surg* 31:330-335, 1973.

32. Eccles JC: Ionic mechanisms of post-synaptic inhibition. *Science* 145:1140, 1964.

33. Sax H, Pletcher J: Local anesthetics: significance of hydrogen bonding in mechanism of action, *Science* 166:1546-1547, 1969.

34. Gissen AJ, Covino BG, Gregus J: Differential sensitivities of mammalian nerve fibers to local anesthetic agents, *Anesthesiology* 53:467-474, 1980.

35. Yagiella JA: Local anesthetics: a century of progress, *Anesth Prog* 32(2):47-56, 1985.

36. Epstein S: Clinical study of prilocaine with varying concentration of epinephrine, *J Am Dent Assoc* 78(1):86-90, 1969.

37. Chilton NW: Clinical evaluation of prilocaine hydrochloride 4% solution with and without epinephrine, *J Am Dent Assoc* 83(2):149-154, 1971.

38. Trieger N, Gillen GH: Bupivacaine anesthesia and postoperative analgesia in oral surgery, *Anesth Prog* 26:20-23, 1979.

39. Chapman PJ, Macleod AWG: A clinical study of bupivacaine for mandibular anesthesia in oral surgery, *Anesth Prog* 32(2):69-72, 1985.

40. Clarkson SW, Hondeghem LM: Mechanism for bupivacaine depression of cardiac conduction: fast block of sodium channels during action potential with slow recovery from block during diastole, *Anesthesiology* 62(4):396-405, 1985.

41. Davis WM Jr, Oakley J, Smith E: Comparison of the effectiveness of etidocaine and lidocaine as local anesthetic agents during oral surgery, *Anesth Prog* 31(4):159-164, 1984.

42. Danielsson K, Evers H, Nordenram A: Long-acting local anesthetics in oral surgery: an experimental evaluation of bupivacaine and etidocaine for oral infiltration anesthesia, *Anesth Prog* 32(2):65-68, 1985.

43. Shannon IL, Feller RP: Contamination of local anesthetic carpules by storage in alcohol, *Anesth Prog* 19(1):6-8, 1972.

44. Aldrete JA, Johnson DA: Allergy to local anesthetics, *J AM Med Assoc* 207(2):356-357, 1969.

45. Malamed SF: Diphenhydramine hydrochloride: its use as a local anesthetic in dentistry, *Anesth Prog* 20:76-81, 1973.

46. Kennett S, Curran JB, Jenkins GR: Management of a broken hypodermic needle: report of a case, *Anesth Prog* 20(2):48-50, 1973.

47. Menke RA, Gowgiel JM: Short-needle block anesthesia at the mandibular foramen, *J Am Dent Assoc* 99:27-30, 1979.

48. Fuller NP, Menke RA, Meyers WJ: Perception of pain to three different intraoral penetrations of needles, *J Am Dent Assoc* 99:822-824, 1979.

49. Trieger N: Anesthetic management of hemophilic during dental treatment. Proceedings of the Dental Hemophilia Institute. University of North Carolina, Chapel Hill, January 1968.

50. Trieger N: *Hemorrhage and hemostasis.* In Guralnick WC, editor: *Textbook of oral surgery,* Boston, 1968, Little, Brown, & Co.

51. Peterson DS, Klein DR: Pain sensation related to local anesthesia injected at varying temperatures, *Anesth Prog* 25(5):164-166, 1978.

52. Dudkiewicz A, Schwartz S, Laliberte R: Effectiveness of mandibular infiltration in children using the local anesthetic Untracaine (articane hydrochloride), *Can Dent Assoc J* 53:29-31, 1987.

53. Lemay H et al: Ultracaine in conventional operative dentistry, *Can Dent Assoc J* 50:703-708, 1984.

5

Premedication: Oral and Intramuscular

Most patients experience a dental visit as an episode of stress, and a small number will demonstrate untoward reactions such as heightened emotional responses, syncope, epileptic seizures, angina pectoris, cardiac dysrhythmias, and even myocardial infarction. Such incidents have been recorded even in the absence of local anesthesia or other medications. What then is the effect of any adjuncts to dental treatment used to allay apprehension, anxiety, and pain? Generally, modalities for controlling pain and anxiety in the dental patient have achieved a high measure of success, although with some attendant complications in a small but significant percentage of patients.

The one common denominator in most complications is the individual patient's physical condition. With careful history and physical evaluation, selection of the most appropriate method of pain and anxiety control for that individual will reduce complications to a minimum. (Special pretreatment medical considerations are discussed in Chapter 3.)

Oral Administration

The list of oral sedative and tranquilizing agents used to secure a more cooperative, conscious patient for dental treatment is extensive. A surprisingly large number of adults come to their appointments fortified with alcohol. Although we may smile or be disconcerted by this, wine and spirits have been used since antiquity to dull perception. The pharmacologic effect of

any drug will depend upon an individual's dose and tolerance. As with most oral sedatives, effects will vary based on the initial level of consciousness and the degree of stress posed by the anticipated procedure, the absorption of the drug from the stomach, the drug content of the blood and brain, and the rate of metabolic breakdown and excretion of the agent.

Oral administration of sedative drugs in the form of pills, capsules, or liquids is usually thought of as the safest route—certainly it is the easiest and most readily accepted by both patient and doctor. It is also, however, one of the least effective and predictable routes of administration. Dosage is usually based on an "average population"—the bell-shaped curve indicating that for a given dose approximately 70% of the population responds in a particular way (one standard deviation from the mean). For the remainder of the group, the dose may be excessive or it may be ineffective. The duration of a drug's effect on that individual may also be of concern. It may wear off too soon or, with some drugs, extend well past the period required and be of potential hazard after the patient leaves the office. Some patients develop a "hangover" after barbiturates. The pharmaceutical literature usually bears a warning advising doctors that their patients should not drive or operate machinery after ingesting these drugs.

Nausea and vomiting may also occur in patients premedicated orally, especially when narcotic analgesics are taken or when the agent causes gastric irritation. Postural hypotension and dizziness too are seen with some agents—in particular, the phenothiazine derivatives. Errors in prescribed dosage are another potential

Portions of this chapter are reprinted, with permission, from Trieger N: Emergencies and complications from sedation modalities," *Dent. Clin. North Am.* 17:3, 1973.

source of hazard and complication, especially with liquid preparations. Zendell reported such an error with a widely used agent, chloral hydrate, in which a child received 10 times the usual dose.[1]

Oral agents are capable of producing allergic reactions in patients previously sensitized. Whereas the delayed type of reaction produces discomfort, the acute anaphylactoid reaction is life-threatening and requires immediate attention. Treatment with epinephrine is indicated in preference to antihistamines. Fortunately, these severe reactions are not common with sedative agents although they are not unknown. A drug history of specific allergies should always be elicited before any drug is prescribed, and every practitioner should be familiar with the recognition and management of these emergencies. Many patients are presently taking a variety of medications chronically: all sedatives and tranquilizers have additive effects to other central nervous system (CNS) depressants, and a number of nonsedative drugs also interact and may produce untoward reactions. Chief among these offenders are the monoamine oxidase (MAO) inhibitors that are used as antidepressant medications. Narcotics given to patients taking MAO inhibitors may precipitate acute hypertensive or hypotensive crises. More is being learned about these areas of drug interaction, and doctors should be aware of the potential for these effects in their patients. Again, a careful preoperative history is essential.

Drug Dosage

Dr. Wayne Hiatt of Ohio State University compares estimating oral and intramuscular drug dosage to the task of an artillery officer who must zero in on his target for maximum effectiveness.[2] His first salvo may be short or long, and he must make the necessary corrections to be exactly on target. Unfortunately, the dentist never has the opportunity to retrieve medication once it is administered and absorbed, and only rarely can a first dose be supplemented to enhance the drug's effect. This would require an additional 30 minutes' waiting period and may still be subject to the same indecisive results. So

the patient may end up undermedicated, appropriately sedated, or overmedicated and depressed.

There are several guides available to estimate appropriate drug dosage, especially for children, but none is entirely satisfactory. In general, careful observation of the patient and individualization of the therapy are essential. Shirkey prefers the use of body surface area calculated from the West nomogram.[3]

$$\frac{\text{Surface area of patient in square meters}}{1.7} \times \text{Adult dose}$$
$$= \text{Approximate dose for child}$$

Clarke's rule is used to estimate the dosage based on the child's weight:

$$\frac{\text{Patient's weight in pounds}}{150} \times \text{Adult dose}$$
$$= \text{Approximate dose for child}$$

Dilling's rule, recommended by Hagen,[4] is based on the patient's age:

$$\frac{\text{Patient's age}}{20} = \text{Fraction of adult dose}$$

The advantages of oral premedication include its simplicity and convenience and the fact that no special equipment or professional attention, other than its initial prescription, is required. It may be better tolerated than injections or an anesthetic mask. It also serves to enhance rapport between dentist and patient by indicating that the doctor is aware and concerned for the safety and comfort of the patient. An important additional placebo effect is not to be denied; Merin[5] and others have shown that the placebo effect is omnipresent.

Intramuscular Administration

Potential problems that may develop with the intramuscular route for sedative drugs include improper dosage or overdosage, hypersensitivity, idiosyncratic reactions, hematomas, nerve injury, and localized sepsis from contaminated equipment.

Anatomic consideration is important in the administration of intramuscular medication if vital nerves are to be avoided. In the upper arm the deltoid muscle is a preferred site of injection. The anterior branch of the axillary nerve winds its way from lateral to medial just inferior to the belly of the muscle. It is deeply situated, against bone. The muscle is grasped and lifted laterally away from the humerus and the injection made slowly, after aspiration, into its bulk.

The gluteal injection is made in the upper outer quadrant of the buttock to avoid the large sciatic nerve trunk. Generally, this should be above an imaginary line drawn from the posterior superior iliac spine to the greater trochanter of the femur. Some authorities recommend the gluteal injections not to be used in young children because they have only thin layers of subcutaneous tissue and muscle; the lateral aspect of the upper thigh is the preferred site in these young children.[6] All injections require aspiration prior to instilling the medication to avoid intravascular injections. Although intramuscular premedication is extensively used prior to general anesthesia in the hospitalized patient, it finds limited use in the dental office. Unlike the hospitalized patient, the office patient must be alert and ambulatory shortly after the end of the dental appointment. Shorter-acting agents are therefore preferable to those usually recommended for preanesthetic medication in the hospital.

The intramuscular route of administration ensures that the patient receives the drug. Vagaries of gastric absorption are bypassed. The onset of action is therefore more predictable. Few patients object to an intramuscular injection, and acceptance is greater than for oral injections. Dosage must be calculated in advance and is therefore inexact when related to a specific individual. Again, as with oral premedication, retrieval of an injected drug is impossible and underdosage rarely merits reinjection within the time available for the appointment.

Patients receiving medications should be warned of their prolonged effects and should avoid taking alcohol or other CNS depressants following the dental appointments. Hypotension, disorientation, agitation, somnolence, dizziness, nausea, and even depression may become manifest following oral or intramuscular medication. The patient should be encouraged to go directly home in the company of a responsible adult and to avoid driving, operating machinery, or even making significant decisions for the remainder of the day. He or she should be encouraged to relax and sleep off the effects of the drug. Baird and Hailey have disclosed an unexplained rise in the plasma level of diazepam 6 hours after its oral ingestion with a recurrence of lassitude.[7]

Tranquilizing and Sedative Drugs

Although many agents have been used for premedication, the special circumstances related to the dental visit preclude the use of very long-acting drugs and those that produce profound depressant effects. Whether given by mouth or by the intramuscular route, dosage for most sedative agents is comparable. Drowsiness and ataxia are infrequently seen in elderly and debilitated patients. The dosage should be decreased for elderly patients and may need to be increased to effect tranquilization in healthy adolescents.

A few of the more commonly used agents are discussed.

Benzodiazepines These agents produce tranquilization, which helps to control the anxiety associated with dental visits. Chlordiazepoxide hydrochloride (Librium) 50 to 100 mg and diazepam (Valium) 5 to 10 mg both effectively reduce excitement and apprehension and can be administered orally or intramuscularly. They do not usually produce the sleepiness or "hangover" associated with the use of barbiturates or other sedative drugs. In addition to their calming action, chlordiazepoxide and diazepam have skeletal muscle relaxant and anticonvulsant effects that have been of help in patients with spastic and convulsive disorders.[7,8] (Triazolam, a newer benzodiazepine recommended for oral sedation in adults is discussed in greater detail at the end of this chapter.)

Anxiety-reducing properties of drugs may either involve or be mediated by the cyclic adenosine monophosphate phosphodiesterase (cyclic AMP) system in the brain. Cyclic AMP, adenyl cyclase (the enzyme that converts adenosine triphosphate [ATP] into cyclic AMP), and cyclic 3',5'—nucleotide phosphodiesterase (the enzyme that hydrolyzes cyclic AMP to 5' AMP) are found in greater abundance in the CNS than in any other tissue. A potent inhibitor of cyclic AMP activity is diazepam. Data indicate that there is a relationship between the effect of a drug on conflict behavior and its ability to inhibit cyclic AMP phosphodiesterase activity in the brain.[9] In this same study, pentobarbital did not inhibit the activity of cyclic AMP phosphodiesterase.

Serotonin antagonists produce anxiety reduction similar to the cyclic AMP phosphodiesterase effects of the benzodiazepines (diazepam) and barbiturates. These drugs decrease the turnover of norepinephrine, serotonin, and other biogenic amines in the brain. This effect may be responsible for some of the behavioral effects of tranquilizers.[10] The primary sites of action of diazepam are said to be the limbic system and those subcortical areas of the brain that are concerned with emotions, that is, midbrain, reticular formation, hypothalamus, and thalamus. Various studies indicate that diazepam blocks pressor responses by a central supraspinal rather than a peripheral mechanism, with a major locus of depressant action in the brainstem reticular system.

Further developments in neuropharmacology have shown specific neurotransmitters and receptors associated with the benzodiazepine drugs. Naturally occurring neurotransmitters such as the amino acid glycine and gamma-aminobutyric acid (GABA) inhibit neurotransmission at specific receptor sites in the CNS. The benzodiazepines enhance the affinity of these neuromodulators for their receptors. The benzodiazepine receptors are located in close proximity to the glycine and GABA-binding sites. Recently, another group of drugs, the imidazobenzepines, has been identified that specifically blocks the binding sites of diazepam without producing any other pharmacologic effects. Flumazenil (Mazicon), available only since 1992, has been successful in reversing overdose of benzodiazepines.[11]

Promethazine Hydrochloride (Phenergan) This agent has pronounced sedative effects and is frequently used for premedication but may be a poor choice for the ambulatory dental patient. Adverse reactions include hypotension and a prolonged duration of effect. It is a phenothiazine and in the same general group of drugs as chlorpromazine hydrochloride (Thorazine). These drugs potentiate other depressants and their adrenergic blocking effects may result in vasodilation and hypotension that does not respond to vasopressors.[12]

Many pediatricians recommend the use of "DPT"(Demerol, Phenergan, and Thorazine) for intramuscular sedation of young children. These drugs are given together, intramuscularly (2 mg/kg, 1 mg/kg, and 1 mg/kg, respectively). This usually produces a very sedated child who, when stimulated, may still be restive and resist dental treatment. The duration of effect of these drugs often persists long after the work is done and may necessitate close attention during the recovery phase.

Hydroxyzine Hydrochloride/Pamoate (Atarax, Vistaril) Hydroxyzine hydrochloride is a useful tranquilizing agent for the dental patient. It also possesses antiemetic and antihistaminic effects. Drowsiness is minimal and transient. This agent has been shown to be teratogenic in animals when given in high dosage: until its role in humans is clarified it should not be used in women of childbearing age. The recommended dosage is 25 mg to 100 mg for adults or 1 mg/kg of body weight for children. It can be given orally in capsule, as a syrup (10 mg/5 ml), in tablet form, or intramuscularly (25 mg/ml).

Secobarbital (Seconal) and Sodium Pentobarbital (Nembutal) Although these drugs are classified as short-acting barbiturates, their actions persist well past the dental appointment. These drugs have been time-tested and do provide sedation and better acceptance of dental treatment by the patient. Untoward effects of the barbiturates are excessive drowsiness, lethargy, and residual sedation ("hangover"). On rare occasions they produce skin eruptions, nausea, and vomiting. Some elderly patients may show a paradoxical restlessness or excitement. These drugs are specifically contraindicated in patients with porphyria, and they should be used with caution in the presence of other depressants and MAO inhibitors.

Barbiturates were widely abused, especially by those habituated to sleep medications and by other dependent individuals. Patients with liver disease (e.g., hepatitis, cirrhosis) should receive reduced dosages. Barbiturates have been described as being antianalgesic with overreaction sometimes precipitated by painful procedures. Nembutal and Seconal are both available in elixirs (2 mg/5 ml), tablets (100 mg), capsules (50 mg), and intramuscular preparations (50 mg/ml). The IM injection should be made deeply within the muscle mass because the high pH of these solutions is irritating.

Meperidine Hydrochloride (Demerol) The need for a narcotic agent in the ambulatory dental patient who receives a local anesthetic to control pain is questionable. Although meperidine hydrochloride has some sedative effect its principal use is as a narcotic analgesic. Particularly in the ambulatory patient, one is likely to encounter adverse side effects such as nausea, vomiting, and hypotension. These are attributable to the blocking of reflexes from receptors in the carotid sinus, aortic arch, and pulmonary vessels, which permit wide fluctuations in blood pressure and the development of orthostatic hypotension when the patient assumes an erect position.[12, 13] Intramuscular meperidine hydrochloride given for postoperative pain relief (75 mg) produced a 60% decrease in pulmonary ventilation within 30 minutes and a 40% change at the end of 2 hours, according to Dripps, Eckenhoff, and Vandam.[14] In a study by Dundee and Clarke[15] patients who received only 100 mg of meperidine hydrochloride for preanesthetic medication exhibited a very high incidence of preoperative nausea and vomiting (34% and 12% respectively). These untoward effects were markedly reduced by giving atropine or scopolamine together with the narcotic. Patients with liver disease, pulmonary emphysema, asthma, advanced age, and-or those in poor general health should seldom be given a narcotic for

premedication because of the higher incidence of side effects relating to circulation and respiration.

Meperidine (and narcotics in general) are also contraindicated for patients receiving MAO inhibitors. They should be used with caution in patients taking other CNS depressants. Demerol is available in tablets (50 mg), as an elixir (50 mg/5 ml), and for injection (50 mg/ml).

There are no specific antidotes for the barbiturates. There is however a specific antagonist that reverses the effects of meperidine. Naloxone hydrochloride (Narcan) does not produce respiratory depression, psychomimetic effects, or pupillary constriction. In the absence of narcotics it shows essentially no pharmacologic activity. To reverse a narcotic's effect, 1 ml (0.4 mg) may be injected intravenously, intramuscularly, or subcutaneously and repeated at 10-minute intervals, as necessary. Benzodiazepines are reversed by injection of flumazenil, recently introduced and very expensive.

Various drug combinations, although widely used, may present some difficulties and potential hazards, especially for the dentist who is inadequately prepared to manage adverse reactions. Most sedative medications are additive or synergistic in effect. All dentists should be knowledgeable and prepared with proper resuscitative equipment to manage untoward reactions in the dental office. These potential catastrophes are not limited to patients receiving adjunctive medication but may occur even in the patient receiving local anesthesia.

Chloral Hydrate Chloral hydrate, one of the oldest sedative drugs, has been extensively used for pediatric patient management. Dosage schedules are usually adjusted from the adult hypnotic range of 500 mg to 1000 mg to lower doses based on the patient's age, weight, body surface area, temperament, and degree of sedation required. It is, fortunately, a forgiving drug—one with a wide safety margin, provided necessary supportive care is given to a patient who is inadvertently oversedated.

It is usually administered as a syrup or elixir, generally in a 500 mg/5 ml (or per tsp). It is important to be familiar with the specific formulation and to calculate dosage in milligram amounts rather than by volume in milliliters, to avoid errors in administration.

Solutions of chloral hydrate are irritating to the gastric mucosa and may induce vomiting. The medication should be followed by water or juice. Recently, concern about the question of tumorogenicity of chloral hydrate has led to a decreased availability and use in clinical practice.

Chloral hydrate is rapidly absorbed and is metabolized in the liver to trichloroethanol. When used in combination with other CNS depressants, the dose administered should be decreased to avoid oversedation. Moore reports that younger children medicated with chloral hydrate and then given nitrous oxide developed airway obstruction.[16] He also cautions about the anesthetics administered to younger children when thoughtful consideration is not given to decreasing dosage according to the weight of the child.

At the present time, in the United States, liability insurance premiums have risen sharply; prompting many dentists to forego the use of intravenous conscious sedation and general anesthesia. Instead, they are trying to make do with oral premedication and sedation. This does not necessarily lead to safer sedation but rather to *less* control of the effects of drugs and even a false sense of security about the patient's well-being.

Regardless of the route of drug administration, the patient must be monitored and vital signs checked repeatedly. The doctor and the office personnel must be appropriately prepared and versed in the management of untoward reactions such as inadvertent unconsciousness, respiratory depression, hypotension, vomiting with a possibility of aspiration of vomitus into the lungs, hyperexcitability, convulsions, etc. Monitoring may take the form of blood pressure determinations, coupled with some continuous appreciation of the pulse. A precordial stethoscope is inexpensive and serves to monitor both heart beat and respiratory sounds. Noninvasive pulse oximeters are available at reasonable cost and serve to provide a continuous evaluation of oxygen saturation—an important early indicator

of hypoxia and impending cardiac dysrhythmias. For most sedation procedures, the use of an electrocardioscope is not advised, unless one is dealing with a medically compromised patient. Such a patient should probably be treated in a hospital or referred for special care.

The appropriate treatment of untoward reactions generally requires the availability of oxygen and a means of delivering positive pressure ventilation. It is not expected that one untrained in general anesthesia techniques should be able to intubate a patient under these difficult circumstances. It is far better to be well versed in maintaining an open airway by proper positioning of the unconscious patient while supplementing the breathing with oxygen and summoning help from the emergency medical service in the local community.

In children, high drug dosage and drug interaction were found to be the principal factors contributing to serious drug reactions, according to Goodson and Moore.[17]

Belladonna Alkaloids Atropine or scopolamine is frequently used in dentistry to reduce excessive salivation and facilitate treatment. In addition, while atropine sulfate (0.4 to 0.6 mg) produces a tachycardia, scopolamine hydrobromide (0.4 mg) produces sedation and dissociation. A higher incidence of excitatory phenomena in those patients receiving scopolamine was reported.[14] The usual doses of these anticholinergic drugs do not increase intraocular pressure even in patients with glaucoma, contrary to popular belief.[12]

Glycopyrrolate (Robinul) is another anticholinergic agent that produces a drying effect. Following intramuscular injection, it works within 10 to 15 minutes but has a protracted effect that lasts for 6 to 7 hours. Of some distinct advantage is the fact that glycopyrrolate does not cause psychomimetic effects or sedation, and although it is vagolytic in action (like atropine and scopolamine), it does not produce a tachycardia. The dosage is 0.2 mg intramuscularly (equivalent to 0.4 mg of atropine) for the adult patient.[18]

Oral midazolam (Versed) is now available in the United States, its use as premedication prior to intravenous sedation is reported from New Zealand.[19] Oral midazolam after 1 hour caused significant anxiety relief and impairment of memory but did not adversely affect postoperative recovery.

Another benzodiazepine, triazolam (Halcion), given preoperatively by mouth, reduced anxiety in a manner comparable to that achieved by intravenous diazepam.[20] This study was done in adult patients undergoing wisdom teeth removal. Triazolam has a 1.5 to 5.5 hour half-life, peaking at 2 hours after ingestion. It has not been approved for use in patients younger than 18 years.

Intramuscular premedication with triazolam compared to diazepam and placebo was studied by Baughman et al.[21] They found that only 0.5 mg of triazolam had a significant effect in reducing anxiety, which was comparable to 15 mg of diazepam. Significant amnesia was also found with 0.5 mg of triazolam, and was greater than that noted with diazepam. However, caution is advised because of some of the side effects noted previously when triazolam was extensively used to treat insomnia. Numerous case reports were cited of amnesia, delirium, psychotic symptoms, anxiety states, and withdrawal difficulties.[22]

Summary

The management of the ambulatory dental patients is often facilitated by the use of oral or intramuscular premedication. The dentist must consider some of the conditions that are unique to the dental office visit, in addition to the uniqueness of the patient's medical and emotional status, when prescribing premedication. The "average" dose is often inadequate for the patient confronted by the stress of anticipated dental treatment. Yet the average patient may be overmedicated by a greater dosage of premedicant. Although oral and intramuscular routes of administration do not allow sufficient flexibility or accuracy to be recommended as primary choices for pain and anxiety control for the office dental patient, they do enhance patient comfort by both pharmacologic and psychologic mechanisms and are widely used.

The effects of premedication frequently outlast the time required for the dental visit, and patients should be advised to avoid posttreatment activities that require attentiveness and coordination, such as automobile driving.

The aim of premedication for dental treatment should be to allay anxiety rather than promote sleepiness or analgesia. For this effect, the tranquilizer Valium is to be recommended over the barbiturates (Nembutal, Seconal) and the narcotics (Demerol).

References

1. Zendell E: Chloral hydrate overdose—a case report, *Anesth Prog* 19:6, 1972.
2. Dr. Wayne Hiatt, Ohio State University: Personal communication, September, 1971.
3. Shirkey HC: General considerations in the care of sick children. In Nelson WE et al, editors: *Textbook of pediatrics,* ed 9, Philadelphia, 1969, WB Saunders, pp. 236-237.
4. Hagen J, Malamed SF, McCarthy FM: *Emergencies in dental practice: prevention and treatment,* ed 2, Philadelphia, 1979, WB Saunders.
5. Merin R: Placebo pharmacology, *Anesth Prog* 20:83-86, 1973.
6. Martin WW et al: *Hazards of medication: a manual of drug interactions, incompatibilities, contraindications, and adverse effects,* Philadelphia, 1971, JB Lippincott.
7. Baird ES, Hailey DM: Delayed recovery from a sedative: correlation of the plasma levels of diazepam with clinical effects after oral and intravenous administration, *Br J Anaesth* 4:803, 1972.
8. deJong RH, Heavner JE: Diazepam prevents local anesthetic seizures, *Anesthesiology* 34:6, 1971.
9. Beer B et al: Cyclic adenosine monophosphate diesterase in brain: effect on anxiety, *Science* 176:428-430, 1972.
10. Wise CD, Berger BD, Stein L: Benzodiazepines: anxiety-reducing activity by reduction of serotonin turnover in the brain, *Science* 177:180-183, 1972.
11. Geller E et al: The use of RO 15-1788: a benzodiazepine antagonist in the diagnosis and treatment of benzodiazepine overdose, *Anesthesiology* 61(3A):A135, 1984.
12. American Medical Association: *American Medical Association Drug Evaluations,* ed 1,

Chicago, 1971, American Medical Association.

13. Friend DG, McLemore GA: Medical progress: some abuses of drugs in therapy, *N Eng J Med* 254(6):1223-1230, 1956.

14. Dripps RD, Eckenhoff JE, Vandam LD: *Introduction to anesthesia,* ed 3, Philadelphia, 1967, WB Saunders.

15. Dundee JW, Clarke RSJ: Studies on atropine, hyoscine and meperidine as preanesthetic medication, *J Oral Ther Pharm* 2(5):386-387, 1966.

16. Moore PA: Pediatric sedation and anesthesia: monitoring and management considerations. Consensus Conference on Anesthesia and Sedation in the Dental Office, April 1985, National Institutes of Health, Bethesda, Md.

17. Goodson MJ, and Moore PA: Life-threatening reactions after pedodontic sedation: an assessment of narcotic, local anesthetic, and antiemetic drug interaction, *J Am Dent Assoc* 107:239-245, 1983.

18. Malamed SF: *Sedation—a guide to patient management,* St Louis, 1989, Mosby Year Book.

19. Luyk NH: Oral midazolam prior to intravenous sedation for the removal of third molars, *J Oral Maxillofac Surg (Suppl)* 48:8, 1:125, 1990.

20. Dionne R, Kaufman E, Hargreaves K: Evaluation of oral triazolam and nitrous oxide for outpatient premedication, *J Dent Res* 69:277, 1990.

21. Baughman V, Becker GL, Ryan CM, Glaser M, Abenstein JP: Effectiveness of triazolam, diazepam, and placebo as preanesthetic medications, *Anesthesiology* 71:196-200, 1989.

22. Kales A: Diagnosis and managment of insomnia, *N Eng J Med* 323:486, 1990 (letter).

6

Nitrous Oxide Psychosedation

Psychosedation with nitrous oxide and oxygen offers an approved approach to patient management for dental treatment. Properly administered, it can be an important adjunct for the control of anxiety in the conscious patient. This is accomplished through the action on the central nervous system (CNS) of the inhalation of controlled amounts of nitrous oxide and oxygen and by its potent placebo effect. Research has demonstrated that it diminishes sensitivity to noxious stimuli in the conscious and responsive patient even in the absence of true analgesia.[1] It is not, however, a substitute for a local analgesic when the procedure is a painful one, or for a full general anesthetic when an unconscious patient is required.

Nitrous oxide–oxygen psychosedation is used in dentistry for a variety of purposes: to aid in radiographic surveys, prophylaxes, and impression taking; to effectively reduce gagging; and to provide a more cooperative patient. Suture removal, changing dressings and packs, wire and splint removal, and cementation of crowns may be carried out more comfortably on the patient sedated with nitrous oxide–oxygen. Operative dentistry, crown and bridge, and nonsurgical periodontics can be performed with the aid of nitrous oxide–oxygen, though it is important to use local analgesia when the operation is anticipated to be a painful one. Extractions and periodontal surgery would generally require adjunctive local analgesia.

The principal advantage to the use of nitrous oxide–oxygen is its rapidity of onset and recovery. With none of the other sedation or anesthesia techniques is there a return to normal as rapidly (120 to 180 seconds) as at the conclusion of nitrous oxide–oxygen psychosedation.[2] The American Dental Association's Council on Dental Therapeutics finds: "In degree of effectiveness, nitrous oxide–oxygen psychosedation is considerably more reliable than the oral route (barbiturates, antianxiety agents), but is equaled or is surpassed by the intravenous route. . . ."[3]

Safety of Use

The record of safety experienced in the use of nitrous oxide–oxygen for conscious patients, in the manner to be detailed, is remarkable. No serious complications have been reported in the performance of many millions of such cases in the past few years. Ruben, in a Danish dental study in 1966, cited the administration of over 3,000,000 sedations without mishap.[4] Important consideration must be given to the concentration of oxygen in this technique. Psychosedation can be achieved and adequate oxygenation ensured if the concentration of oxygen is never lower than 25%. More often a 50% concentration of oxygen is used for satisfactory sedation with nitrous oxide. Nitrous oxide depresses bone marrow and peripheral white blood cell counts after prolonged use, that is, more than 48 hours of continuous use. However, its administration as a sedative agent in the manner in which it is generally used has failed to demonstrate any toxic effect.

Jaffe, in a searching paper, reviewed the literature and concluded that, "Nitrous oxide used properly is still the least toxic of all anes-

Portions of this chapter have been reprinted from Trieger N, Carr W: Psychosedation. In McCarthy FM, editor: *Emergencies in dental practice, prevention and treatment,* ed 2, Philadelphia, 1972, WB Saunders.

75

thetic agents".[5] Everett and Allen report that the cardiorespiratory effects of nitrous oxide–oxygen sedation (with nitrous oxide given in concentrations of up to 40%) parallel those of inhaling 100% oxygen.[6,7] The changes in cardiac output and total peripheral resistance are small and inconsequential. Wynne et al also found that nitrous oxide inhalation in patients undergoing cardiac catheterization does not produce important depression of left ventricular performance.[8] Eisele et al had previously found that 40% nitrous oxide inhalation depresses myocardial function in patients with coronary occlusion and left ventricular dysfunction.[9] When used to supplement other inhalation anesthetics, nitrous oxide has depressive as well as stimulatory effects, depending on the dosage used as well as the primary anesthetic employed.[10] Philbin et al found a direct detrimental effect on areas of the myocardium supplied by a compromised coronary artery when nitrous oxide was used in conjunction with the intravenous narcotic fentanyl citrate.[11]

In the last decade important new data have been published showing that nitrous oxide is neither inert nor innocuous when inhaled. Prolonged exposure to even low doses has been associated with a higher incidence of spontaneous abortion and liver disease (even after excluding serum hepatitis).[12,13] In rats nitrous oxide has been shown to induce infertility by disruption of hypothalamic cells, which produce hormone-releasing hormone.[14]

After further study and surveys of populations at risk, the United States National Institute for Occupational Safety and Health recommended that 30 ppm of nitrous oxide or less is a "tolerable" level in the operating room.

Nunn and Chanarin point out that nitrous oxide inactivates the vitamin B_{12} (cobalamin or methylcobalamin) component of the enzyme methionine synthetase.[15] DNA synthesis is thus impaired, producing delayed red blood cell maturation and leucopenia when inhalation lasts longer than 24 hours.

Neurotoxicity from the abuse of nitrous oxide has been reported.[16,17] The clinical signs and symptoms were similar to those of subacute combined degeneration of the spinal cord seen in vitamin B_{12} deficiency. Recovery followed slowly after the abuse was discontinued. Nunn also indicates that while a nitrous oxide anesthetic "of even moderate length" produces inhibition of methionine and DNA synthesis, "billions of patients have breathed nitrous oxide without apparent harm."[15] His studies show that operating room staff exposed to concentrations between 200 and 400 ppm have normal serum methionine levels. He finds "nonconvincing evidence to support the recommendation of the National Institute for Occupational Safety and Health of a time-weighted average of 25 ppm."[15] Nevertheless, the use of scavenging of waste gases and other techniques to minimize pollution is highly recommended. These will be discussed in the section on equipment.

Malignant hyperpyrexia has been reported in association with nitrous oxide use.[18] It is believed to be only an indirect effect, perhaps contributing to the problem by increasing sympathetic activity and heat production.

Psychologic studies of human performance during exposure to nitrous oxide (500 ppm) and enflurane (15 ppm) were reported by Bruce and Bach[19] and also for nitrous oxide (50 ppm) and halothane (1 ppm).[20] They found measurable decrements in performance of some psychologic tests involving visual perception, immediate memory, and a combination of perception, cognition, and motor response. These changes were not found when subjects were exposed to 25 ppm nitrous oxide and 0.5 ppm halothane. Subsequent studies do *not* confirm the earlier findings of impairment. Higher percentages (20% to 30%) of nitrous oxide are required to produce these adverse effects—at levels "200 to 400 times greater than the average levels found in nonscavenged operating rooms."[21]

Cautions and Contraindications

There are two primary potential problems to consider—hypoxia and excitement. Hypoxia can be avoided by adequate oxygen flow. Newer machines provide a delivery system that requires a minimum of 25% to 30% oxygen before the nitrous oxide will flow. This serves as an important safeguard, provided the system has been properly hooked up and oxygen is being fed to the oxygen inlet.

Excitement can be prevented by avoiding too deep a sedation, which may readily change to the excitement stage of general anesthesia. Certain machines are designed to provide a maximum of 50% nitrous oxide. Others are set to permit a maximum of 70% nitrous oxide. There are few contraindications to the use of nitrous oxide–oxygen sedation. There are, however, significant contraindications for elective treatment given to certain patients with significant health problems. Patients with congestive heart failure who are decompensated should not receive elective dental treatment. The rendering of emergency care to relieve pain and infection may become necessary. Similarly, patients who have sustained a myocardial infarction in the past 6 months should have all elective work deferred. Patients with advanced pulmonary disease (e.g., emphysema) are also poor candidates for anesthesia.

However, these patients, as well as those with congestive heart failure and recent myocardial infarction, may benefit by the administration of oxygen during the performance of essential dental work. This often serves to provide an enriched oxygen atmosphere and aids to decrease anxiety and provide better tissue perfusion. The dentist must be aware of the possibility of producing adverse effects in the patient with advanced emphysema. Some of these patients, because of poor diffusion, have built up carbon dioxide blood levels that exceed normal and no longer provide the normal drive for respiration. Instead, lowered blood oxygen levels are responsible for the respiratory drive. Providing too much oxygen to these patients (in excess of 24% to 28%) may produce respiratory arrest. Patients with severe anemia may benefit from the adjunctive administration of high levels of oxygen, but should not be made to undergo anesthesia or other treatment that further depresses the oxygen-carrying capacity of the blood or cardiac function.

Nasal obstruction, upper respiratory infec-

tions, and allergic rhinitis are considered important contraindications for nitrous oxide–oxygen sedation. We are dependent upon the nasal airway, and patients who have significant nasal obstruction will not be able to benefit from this technique.

Patients receiving monoamine oxidase (MAO) inhibitors (such as Nardil, Marplan, Parnate, Eutonyl), which are generally prescribed for emotional antidepressive effects, and those receiving cortisone or related steroid medications are particularly susceptible to the hazards associated with stress and anesthesia.

One of the most significant contraindications to the use of nitrous oxide–oxygen psychosedation is emotional instability. Because this method causes some distortion of normal perception, it would be unwise to involve schizoid patients. It is undoubtedly far better when dealing with patients who are emotionally disturbed to maintain their tenuous contact with the reality of the treatment situation.

Pregnancy, especially the first trimester, has been cited as a contraindication for nitrous oxide–oxygen psychosedation.[7,15] Baden reports that there is little reason to believe that nitrous oxide is mutagenic;[22] however, animal studies have shown adverse reproductive effects. Epidemiologic studies show an increased incidence of spontaneous abortion in women exposed to waste anesthetic gases, especially nitrous oxide.

Pretreatment patient evaluation is essential to avoid potential complications. The reader is referred to Chapter 3 for a more detailed consideration of this topic.

Nitrous Oxide Induction

The initial absorption of nitrous oxide is extremely rapid. Approximately 1000 ml at a normal respiratory minute volume is taken up within the first minute. At the end of 10 minutes, it drops to 350 ml, in 30 minutes it drops further to 200 ml, and drops to only 100 ml in 100 minutes. Studies by Eger, Saidman, and Brandstater show that breathing 100% nitrous oxide takes only 1 minute to reach 80% alveolar concentration.[23] At 1% nitrous oxide it takes 4 to 5

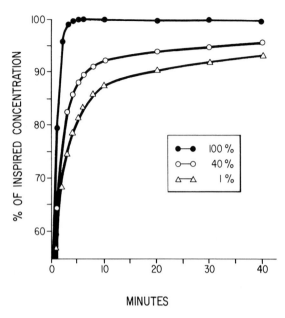

Fig. 6-1. Alveolar concentration of nitrous oxide rapidly approaches the inspired concentration. (From Eger EI: Uptake, distribution and elimination of nitrous oxide. In Hustead RF, Eastwood DW, editors: *Clinical anesthesia—nitrous oxide,* Philadelphia, 1964, FA Davis.)

minutes to reach 80% of that inspired concentration (Fig. 6-1).

It is readily demonstrable that it generally takes approximately 40 seconds of breathing nitrous oxide for patients to experience sensory changes such as tingling, feeling "high," feeling warmth, and other changes in perception. Hustead and Eastwood have demonstrated, in the use of nitrous oxide for obstetrics, that when pain is present during labor, only 30% of patients reported decrease in pain with the administration of nitrous oxide–oxygen sedation.[24] This percentage increased significantly when labor pains were of short duration, patients apparently having confidence that the gas helped to relieve their discomfort. Nitrous oxide is rapidly transmitted to the fetus across the placenta but does not influence uterine contraction.[25] This strongly suggests an important placebo effect in the control of pain.

Patient response to nitrous oxide varies greatly. Patient must provide their own titration. There can be no arbitrary or predetermined levels because we are dealing with individuals who differ enormously in their response to the percentage of nitrous oxide.

The position of the patient is also an important consideration. Elevation of the legs, as is customarily practiced in contour dental chairs, will diminish the likelihood of blood pooling in the lower extremities. Patients with cardiopulmonary disease generally have the greatest lung compliance in the sitting position. A combination of legs up and the head and thorax at a 30-degree angle is often practiced and may overcome some of the problems of patient positioning.

Induction of anesthesia is dependent upon the partial pressure of the gas, its solubility (i.e., rate of uptake by blood and then by tissues), and its potency. In consideration of the pulmonary factor, a primary point is the rate of ventilation, which determines the early uptake. Thus, breath holding would certainly delay the onset of the anesthetic effect, and rapid deep breathing would tend to increase the rate of uptake. Transfer of the gas from the pulmonary alveoli to the blood is dependent upon its rate of diffusion. Diffusion is a function of its solubility, the rate of pulmonary blood flow (i.e, cardiac output), and the tension of the gas in the arterial and venous blood. Further, the blood-to-tissue transfer is dependent upon the following:

1. Solubility of the gas in the tissues. With nitrous oxide, blood and tissue solubility (except for fat) are almost the same. (Nitrous oxide is relatively insoluble when compared to other inhalation anesthetics.)

2. The rate of blood flow for perfusion of the tissues. In this regard, the brain's blood supply is many times that of the body, and hence an effect is noted on the CNS very rapidly.

3. The tension of the anesthetic gas. Graphically, the induction of anesthesia may be pictured as a series of swinging doors at the several exchange points. The gas entering into the lungs meets the alveolar

barrier before entering the venous circulation. Once carried by the blood, it is pumped out by the heart to where it encounters the barrier to the tissues.

Characteristics of Nitrous Oxide

Nitrous oxide gas, which is prepared by heating ammonium nitrate, is compressed and liquified in blue cylinders at a pressure of 800 psi. It is stable and does not react with soda lime, which is often used to absorb carbon dioxide during anesthesia. It will support combustion but will not explode or burn. No chemical reaction occurs on inhalation. It is a sweet-tasting gas and not unpleasant to inhale. It is eliminated by the lungs, skin, sweat, urine, and intestinal gas. All modalities of sensation may be affected, depending upon the concentration of gas administered. Acuity of hearing, sight, touch, pain, memory, concentration, and calculation are affected. Electroencephalographic changes are minimal. Cerebellar functions are affected and produce incoordination and psychomotor deficits, ataxia, and nystagmus. Nitrous oxide has a pronounced effect on the sensorium at subanesthetic levels. Changes in heart rate, cardiac output, blood pressure, or central venous pressure are generally insignificant except when approaching the excitement stage of anesthesia.

At subanesthetic concentrations, blood pressure and pulse rate show a gradual and moderate decline that may well be a reflection of the sedation achieved. These reductions in heart rate and blood pressure tend to persist into the recovery even after the patient's sensorimotor changes have been restored to normal.[2] This may account for the postsedation feeling of relaxation. At higher concentrations, nitrous oxide has been found to produce signs of sympathetic activation with increases in cardiovascular parameters.[26] Venodilation of the skin vessels occurs during nitrous oxide administration, and this may facilitate venipuncture. A diaphoresis, or sweating, often occurs with nitrous oxide induction. Belladonna alkaloids (atropine) may help control this phenomenon.

In a laboratory study involving human volunteers, nitrous oxide at 33% was shown to reduce sensitivity to radiant heat as well as the willingness to report pain.[27] In 1976 the "analgesic" effect of nitrous oxide was suggested to resemble an opiate effect and to be responsive, in part, to being blocked by narcotic antagonists such as naloxone hydrochloride.[28] The interaction of nitrous oxide with the opiate receptor–endorphin system is not straightforward.[29] Chen and Quock have suggested that nitrous oxide analgesia involves spinal and supraspinal kappa-opioid but not mu-opioid receptors.[30]

The Psychosedation Technique

It is important that all persons (secretaries, assistants, laboratory technicians, hygienists) employed in the office be made aware of proper office demeanor when a patient is undergoing nitrous oxide–oxygen sedation. The office should have a quiet, relaxed atmosphere prior to and throughout the psychosedation procedure. It is necessary to avoid loud noises or other distractions, such as excessive talking, in the presence of the patient. Remember that the patient under the influence of nitrous oxide–oxygen is conscious but statements made within hearing of the patient may be distorted and misinterpreted.

The duties of the assistant can be accomplished with greater empathy and more efficiency if the assistant has experienced nitrous oxide–oxygen sedation. All personnel involved with patients having this procedure should experience the sensations produced by nitrous oxide, under supervision.

The duties of the dental assistant in regard to the preparation of the patient for nitrous oxide–oxygen sedation begin with an explanation to the patient about the steps that are about to be taken. If the assistant has experienced this method of sedation, he or she can then describe to patients the sensations they will experience. At this point, it is well to avoid unrealistic promises. Avoid telling the patient not to worry; this is an impossible command to comply with and often suggests to the patient that perhaps there is something to be concerned about. The nasal hood is adjusted to ensure comfort during the psychosedation session. Under the dentist's directions, the assistant may regulate the flow of gases.

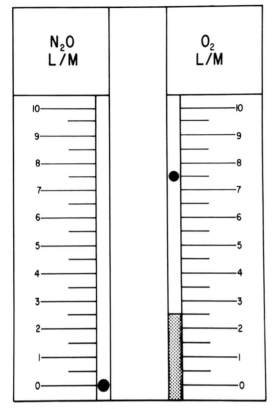

Fig. 6-2. Flowmeters. Oxygen is set first to determine adequacy of total flow.

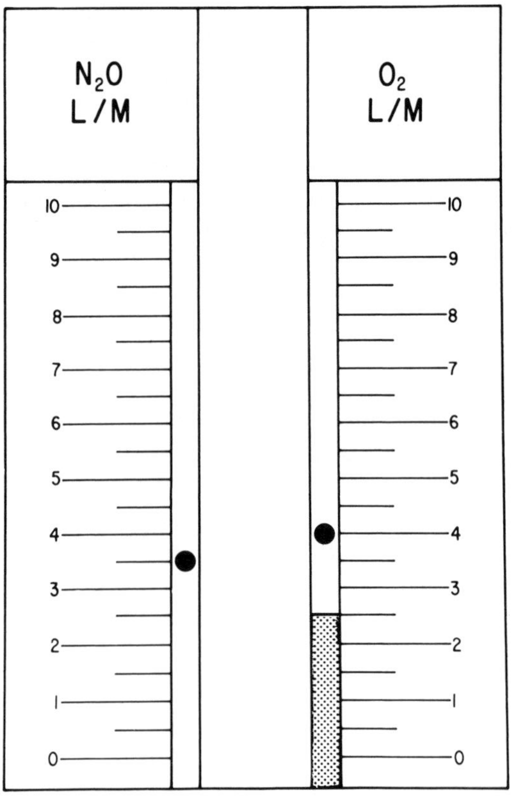

Fig. 6-3. Flowmeters. Achieving "baseline" for psychosedation; individualizing is important.

The procedure has been explained to familiarize the patient with what is about to happen, and the sensations of warmth and tingling he or she will experience are described. The nose mask is adjusted comfortably, and the flow of 4 to 7 L/min of oxygen is continued for 1 to 3 minutes. At this point, the bag should be checked to avoid underinflation or overdistention. The liter flow per minute is determined by our estimate of the patient's tidal flow, based on the size and metabolic rate of the individual (Fig. 6-2). Following this oxygenation period, nitrous oxide is introduced at 1 L/min and oxygen decreased 1 L/min., there should be pause of 30 to 45 seconds at each stop until "baseline" area is achieved. When baseline is achieved for the patient with a 7 L/min flow, the flowmeter might then look like Fig. 6-3.

To determine the actual percentages of gases flowing, the calculations are quite simple. A flow of 3 L/min of nitrous oxide and 4 L/min of oxygen constitutes a 7 L/min total; 3 L/min of nitrous oxide is almost 43% of the total flow, and oxygen at 4 L/min is almost 60%. Generally, 25% to 40% nitrous oxide will be effective in carrying the patient to the level of psychosedation desired.

This technique minimizes the risk of overshooting and precipitating a problem by carrying the patient too deeply into the excitement stage of general anesthesia. Such an event constitutes one of the two principal hazards associ-

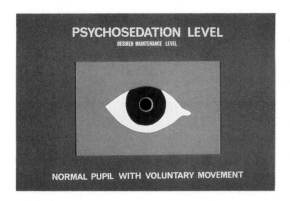

Fig. 6-4. Normal pupil with voluntary movement.

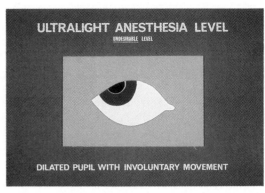

Fig. 6-5. Dilated pupil with involuntary movement.

ated with the administration of nitrous oxide–oxygen sedation. At all times the patient must remain conscious and in contact with the surroundings. The alveolar concentration of nitrous oxide is a function of time as well as administered concentration of gas. At lesser concentration of nitrous oxide, psychosedation will be achieved in a few more minutes. Never give less than 25% oxygen—avoid the other potential hazard, which is that of hypoxia. Modern sedation machines are especially designed to prevent the administration of less than 20% to 25% oxygen. This safeguard is important if we are to avoid hypoxia.

The "baseline" is determined by communicating with the patient. Remember that you are dealing with a conscious patient. Ask the patient, "Do you feel as if you're floating?" "Are you dreaming?" "Are you comfortable?" The patient may respond with hesitation. If the patient is questioned about the hesitation, the reply usually is something like, "I heard you, but it was too much trouble to answer." At this point, the patient's eyes are generally closed and he or she speaks with difficulty. Respiration is normal and there is no holding of breath or grunting. If the patient should slip into deep sedation or ultralight anesthesia, there can be superficial slow breathing, which is often irregular with prolonged inspirations, phonations, and grunting.

Other signs that help us know that we are maintaining our patient in the proper stage are the facial expressions of the conscious individual as compared to facial expressions that represent pain in semiconsciousness. The patient's eyes in the proper stage are also an aid, with normal-sized pupils that contract normally to light. There is no rolling of the eyeballs. If the patient sinks too deeply, the pupils may become dilated and contract actively to light and the eyeballs roam (Figs. 6-4 and 6-5). The pulse rate and blood pressure are not definitive aids in determining the level of sedation. It is our aim to maintain each patient at the proper sedative level (Fig. 6-6, barred zone). Patients who approach the excitement or ultralight anesthesia level can be returned to baseline by decreasing the nitrous oxide and increasing the oxygen flow.

When patients are to have a great deal of dental therapy, it is useful to teach them to lighten the sedation by breathing through their mouths or, if discomfort is experienced, to take deep breaths through the nose to increase the concentration of nitrous oxide being delivered.

At the completion of dental procedures, the nitrous oxide is turned off while the oxygen flow is increased to the original 4 to 7 L/min flow. The oxygen should be continued for approximately 2 minutes or until the effects of the sedation have disappeared. Allow patients to re-

PRE-ANALGESIC STAGE	CONSCIOUS, ORIENTED, ANXIOUS
ANALGESIA-AMNESIA STAGE (DESIRED STAGE)	CONSCIOUS, RELAXED, FLOATING, WARMTH, LESSENED ANXIETY, EUPHORIA
"PRE"-EXCITEMENT and ULTRA-LIGHT ANESTHESIA STAGE	NON-ORIENTED, RESTLESS, HYPERRESPONSIVE TO STIMULI
SURGICAL ANESTHESIA PLANES 1 2 3 RESPIRATORY HAZARD	UNCONSCIOUSNESS (NITROUS OXIDE LACKS POTENCY TO ANESTHETIZE PATIENTS INTO SURGICAL PLANES OF ANESTHESIA)

Fig. 6-6. Schematic of the level desired in relationship to the stages of anesthesia.

main seated until they feel normal. They should never be dismissed if they are still feeling sluggish.

Subjective Reactions

The early subjective symptoms, which are sometimes but not always present, include tingling sensations in the toes, the fingertips, the tip of the tongue, or the lips. These feelings can be readily determined by direct questioning, because we are dealing with a conscious patient. If patients cannot respond to questions, this is a signal that they have sunk below the level of sedation. The operator should immediately decrease the liter flow of nitrous oxide and increase the oxygen by a corresponding amount. Another useful sign of the patient's level is based on his or her ability to maintain the mouth in the open position. For this reason a mouth prop, used routinely for patients who are undergoing a general anesthetic, is *not* recommended. The sedated patient who is being maintained at the proper level can keep the mouth open in a relaxed manner. If the mouth slowly begins to close, this indicates that the nitrous oxide flow should be decreased, with a corresponding increase in the oxygen flow. The total liter flow initially decided as the proper amount (tidal flow) for this patient should be maintained without underinflation or overdistention of the bag.

Another subjective symptom the patient may experience is a warm wave sweeping over the entire body after the initial tingling sensations. A feeling of lethargy and relaxation may be experienced. The occasional patient experiences a humming or vibratory sensation throughout the body, somewhat like a finely tuned motor softly

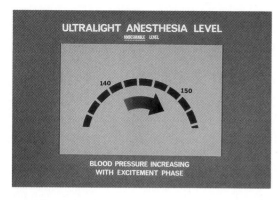

Fig. 6-7. Blood pressure increasing with excitement phase.

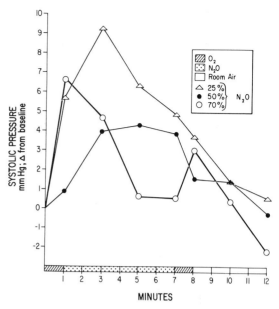

Fig. 6-9. Influence of various concentrations of nitrous oxide on systolic blood pressure.

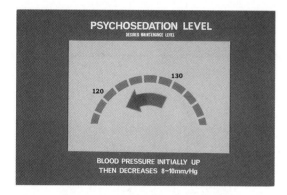

Fig. 6-8. Blood pressure initially up, then decreases 8 to 10 mm Hg.

purring. Patients at the ideal plane for operating often experience a floating sensation. At this point, the baseline is established and the patient maintained at a slightly reduced level of nitrous oxide. This is the ideal time to inject a local anesthetic, because the patient is conscious and responsive to the needle prick but will care less about the discomfort produced.

Objective Reactions

Minor alterations of blood pressure, pulse rate, and respiration are noted in patients undergoing nitrous oxide–oxygen sedation. Blood pressure changes are best illustrated in Figs. 6-7 to 6-11.

Alterations of pulse rate are shown in Figs. 6-12 to 6-14.

Respiration under the desired maintenance level of nitrous oxide–oxygen sedation reflects smooth, regular breathing (Fig. 6-14). When the depth of sedation is increased, respirations become irregular and may be deep or shallow, characteristic of early excitement (Fig. 6-13).

Incoordination becomes evident during inhalation sedation when the patient is requested to perform some specific activity. In a study designed to show the effects of nitrous oxide–oxygen sedation on psychomotor performance,[2] marked changes were demonstrated and related to the depth of sedation. A self-administered, simple line-drawing test was used; patients were asked to connect a series of dots on the test to complete the outline of the figure. A baseline drawing was taken prior to the influence of any agent. The test was then repeated at suitable intervals to determine decrement in performance, as well as recovery to the patient's own baseline. Figure 6-15 demonstrates a composite of several tests administered

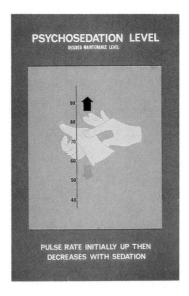

Fig. 6-10. Pulse rate initially up, then decreases with sedation.

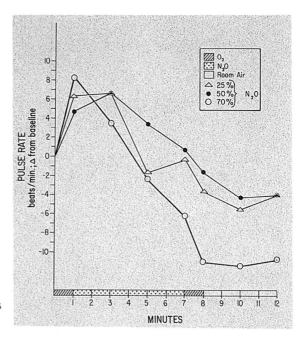

Fig. 6-12. Influence of various concentrations of nitrous oxide on pulse rate.

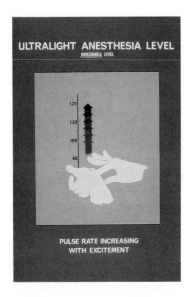

Fig. 6-11. Pulse rate increasing with excitement.

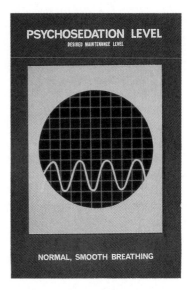

Fig. 6-13. Normal, smooth breathing.

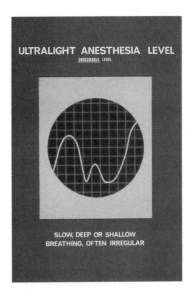

Fig. 6-14. Slow, deep or shallow breathing, often irregular.

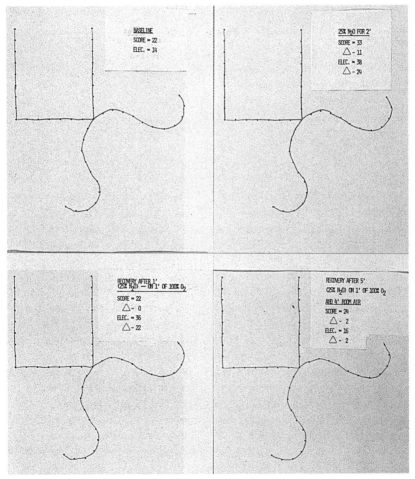

Fig. 6-15. Series of tests by the same subject showing moderate impairment of psychomotor coordination caused by drug effect and recovery.

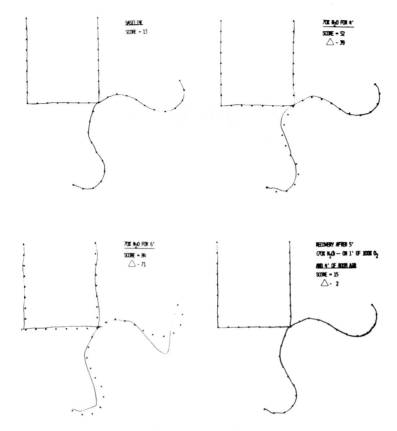

Fig. 6-16. Series of tests showing severe psychomotor incoordination in a patient receiving 70% nitrous oxide.

to the same patient undergoing sedation at a constant percentage of nitrous oxide and oxygen. Figure 6-16 shows a similar series of drawings under a higher concentration of nitrous oxide. In almost all cases studied, return to normal baseline occurs within 2 to 4 minutes after cessation of the nitrous oxide. This test can be numerically scored to yield objective data that can be evaluated by statistical analysis (Fig. 6-17).

Such testing may help in the preanesthetic evaluation of patients. The test is a modification of the Bender Motor Gestalt Test, which has been used extensively to measure psychomotor performance in brain-damaged children.[31]

In this same study,[2] electrical stimulation of the lower lip was used to determine threshold reactions to a noxious stimulus. Although no correlation in this experimental setup can be made to clinical pain situations, results showed an "analgesic" effect attributable largely to placebo influence and less so to the nitrous oxide–oxygen administration (Fig. 6-18). Fig. 6-18 shows almost 5 minutes of breathing 50% nitrous oxide for these uninitiated subjects to reach the level of maximal pain tolerance. The second exposure was to 70% nitrous oxide, and the maximal response came earlier. On the third experience, when these same subjects were no longer naive, they responded within the first minute of only 25% nitrous oxide inhalation with maximal pain tolerance (a beautiful example of the placebo effect.) Despite this rapidly learned response, their pain tolerance declined even though they continued to breathe nitrous

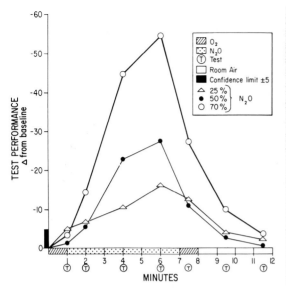

Fig. 6-17. Psychomotor performance modified by three different nitrous oxide concentrations—evaluated by statistical analysis.

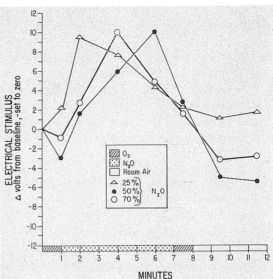

Fig. 6-18. The influence of nitrous oxide on response to electrical stimulation of the lower lip.

oxide–oxygen. Similar responses are common in the treatment situation when the patient continues to feel "at ease" despite the fact that the nitrous oxide concentration has been markedly reduced or even eliminated.

The experienced clinician makes good use of this placebo influence by varying the administration of nitrous oxide throughout the dental procedure. This not only reduces the amount of drug the patient receives but also reduces the cost of administration.

Recovery From Nitrous Oxide

The elimination of nitrous oxide follows a reverse serve pattern of uptake. A large volume is removed initially. This high initial outpouring of nitrous oxide was thought to produce hypoxia (diffusion anoxia) on recovery by displacing oxygen. Though this is not usually found with nitrous oxide–oxygen sedation, following general anesthesia there is a tendency toward hypoventilation on recovery, as carbon dioxide is blown off and the respiratory rate falls. Oxygen administration at the end of each procedure is advis-

able for 2 to 3 minutes after the nitrous oxide is shut off.

Complications

Expectoration Patients should be discouraged from expectorating. This can be accomplished by making liberal use of the aspirator (suction). If it is absolutely necessary for the patient to expectorate, the assistant should place his or her hand as a guide on the patient's forehead to prevent bumping of the patient's head on the cuspidor when the patient is bending over.

Nausea This condition is rare with nitrous oxide sedation, though it may occur with patients who have consumed a heavy meal prior to their dental appointment or have been carried too deeply into the pre-excitement stage. Although we do not usually advise abstinence from food prior to a sedation appointment, it may be necessary to do so with these patients. Some patients who are prone to develop motion sickness may also be more prone to develop nausea.

Vomiting If vomiting occurs, the gas must be discontinued. The nasal mask is removed and the patient tipped forward to allow facilitation of emesis. A high-volume suction evacuator will facilitate removal of vomitus.

Perspiration Usually perspiration can be disregarded unless it is accompanied by pallor and other evidence of cardiovascular distress, such as decrease in blood pressure and increase in pulse rate.

Behavioral Problems Patients who become too deeply anesthetized may develop dissociation, with emotionally disturbing dreams and psychic distortions and reactions. We must guard against this type of untoward reaction and prevent the patient from reaching this stage. Some patients with prior adverse reactions to general and even spinal anesthesia may develop intense anxieties while undergoing the sensory change of nitrous oxide sedation. It is often best to discontinue the administration, allow the patient to discuss the recall of experience, and then, if agreeable, suggest a subsequent opportunity to try it again in the near future. Reassure the patient that he or she can stop the procedure by signaling if this severe anxiety returns and by taking some deep breaths through the mouth. Some patients may resent the threat of feeling "out of control" when they begin to experience subjective tingling, floating, or numbness. These patients are often rigid, "uptight" people. They may reach up and pull off the nasal mask when they feel threatened about their loss of control. Nevertheless, their wishes should be honored, and they should be given time and opportunity to learn how to control their nitrous oxide sedation. Perhaps the greatest harm we can do is to insist on adapting each patient to the same technique instead of adapting a variety of approaches to different patients' needs.

Pressure-Volume Effect As Duncan and Moore point out, nitrous oxide tends to diffuse rapidly into air cavities, displacing nitrogen.[32] The middle ear cavity is most susceptible, and patients receiving nitrous oxide report auditory changes and hearing reduction that is tempo-rary. Minimizing duration and nitrous oxide concentration can reduce these potential pressure/volume problems.

Psychologic Problems Nitrous oxide psychosedation alters the patient's perceptions. Hallucinations have been reported in a very small percentage of patients.[33] Patients who are psychotic are best managed by maintaining their tenuous contact with reality and treated with other sedative and anxiolytic techniques.

One of the most disconcerting aspects of nitrous oxide psychosedation has been the number of complaints of sexual molestation. Misperceptions of "touch" and the intimate nature of the dentist-patient relationships mandate the presence of a third person whenever nitrous oxide sedation is used. *Never* administer a mind-altering drug such as nitrous oxide in the absence of a third person. It is reassuring to the patient and medicolegally essential that the dentist have another person present. Those instances where a patient is under the influence of nitrous oxide and is abused by a dentist are very few compared to the incidence of misperceptions. The only way to avoid such problems is to insist on the presence of a third party.

Adjunctive Drug Therapy

The advantages of rapid onset of sedation and rapid recovery may well be voided by the administration of other drugs orally, intramuscularly, or intravenously. Also, it may confuse the anticipated reactions by the patient. It is best to use nitrous oxide–oxygen sedation with adjunctive local analgesia only.

Experienced operators often combine the techniques of inhalation and intravenous sedation. They induce with nitrous oxide–oxygen and then initiate the intravenous puncture. The nitrous oxide–oxygen is then discontinued, and within 1 to 2 minutes the patient returns to normal. At this time the intravenous medication is titrated and signs and symptoms of its action noted. The nitrous oxide may then be resumed, with the concentration of the gas required at a lower level. Not all patients are appropriate candidates for nitrous oxide sedation. Some will require a complete general anesthetic, whereas others are cooperative with only local analgesia. Each patient must be uniquely evaluated and managed.

It has been recommended that oxygen and a means to efficiently administer it to patients are integral parts of any dentist's armamentarium. The presence of an inhalation sedation machine in the office satisfies this requirement. It can be helpful as an adjunct in the management of many conditions.

Emergencies

Although emergencies are extremely rare with nitrous oxide–oxygen sedation, all members of the dental profession should try to be prepared for any emergency that can occur in the dental office.

Airway Obstruction   Obstruction of the airway through whatever cause demands immediate attention. In this technique of nitrous oxide–oxygen sedation, one is dealing with a conscious patient who responds rapidly to an intrusion threatening the airway. The operator must exercise care in the use of high-speed instrumentation and its copious water flow, with the aid of a high-volume suction in addition to the watchful eyes of the operator and assistant. The airway may be aspirated with tonsil tip suction to evacuate any large quantity of fluid. Additionally, there are a few maneuvers that will very quickly assist in re-establishing a good airway. The simplest of these is to elevate the patient's chin and to hyperextend the neck or pull the mandible forward. The operator may also place his or her forefingers behind the angles of the jaw and push the mandible forward, which will free the airway by simultaneously pulling the tongue and tissues of the floor of the mouth out of the oropharynx.

In the unconscious patient, this simple maneuver will often result in a deep inspiration and the patient's return to consciousness. If respirations are depressed, oxygen should be administered immediately via the nasal mask. The additional attachment of a face mask is important to assist depressed respiration. The use of endotracheal tubes and a laryngoscope requires significant training in anesthesiology and is well beyond the scope of those not trained in general anesthetic techniques.

Apparatus for Psychosedation

Modern machines have been significantly redesigned to enhance the safe administration of nitrous oxide–oxygen. These differ from anesthesia machines and are intended to prevent some of the potential problems inherent in general anesthesia. Most modern sedation units are programmed so that they will not function below 25% oxygen. This is to eliminate the potential hazard of hypoxia. Some machines are programmed to deliver no more than 50% nitrous oxide. This is to minimize overly deep sedation and pre-excitement. All machines now have a "fail-safe" oxygen system. Should the supply of oxygen drop, the nitrous oxide flow automatically discontinues. Some machines also incorporate an audible signal to alert the operator that the fail-safe has been activated.

The term *inhalation sedation unit* is preferred to the term *analgesia unit* because it would properly emphasize the aim of this technique, which is to achieve sedation and relaxation of the conscious patient. This unit should be a continuous flow machine. Our own experience, as well as studies by McCarthy and Shuken[34] and Allen, Gehrig, and Tolas[35] proves that the demand flow unit is not as efficient and in some cases is unsafe, whereas the continuous flow unit is efficient, safe, and ideal for this technique. The relative accuracy of the continuous flow unit is an acknowledged fact.

The gases in a continuous flow machine move continually at the rates set on the flowmeters and are not related to the patient's respirations. The demand flow machine, also called the *on-demand* or *intermittent flow machine,* does not flow continually at a set rate. The dial is set at a given percentage for the proportions of the two gases, and the output responds and varies with the patient's respiratory needs.

Continuous flow inhalation sedation units

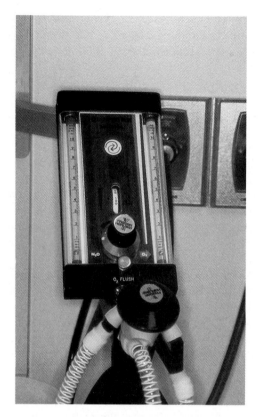

Fig. 6-19. Psychosedation unit permitting a maximum of 50% nitrous oxide and equipped with antipollution mask.

can be of the portable cylinder type or part of a permanent installation system. Those units that are part of an installed system can be wall mounted, stand mounted, or cabinet mounted. This flexibility permits greater convenience in introducing an inhalation sedation unit into the office.

Flowmeters that record the flow of gases in liters per minute should be readily visible. They operate simply by having a small ball within the transparent flow tube floating on the column of flowing gas. The greater the flow, the higher the ball floats. The push-button direct oxygen flush bypasses the regular flowmeters, providing a minimal flow of 30 L/min of oxygen into the mask. This is for use in an emergency to fill the bag or whenever a sudden increase in oxygen is desirable.

Reservoir (Rebreathing) Bags   These are available in a variety of sizes from 1 to 8 liters. The 3- and 5-L sizes are most commonly used. It is essential that the unit have a reservoir bag for several reasons. In the technique advocated, observation of the bag gives the operator an accurate guide to the patient's tidal flow. It is particularly important that the inhalation sedation unit have a bag in the breathing circle for certain emergencies. Positive pressure oxygen can be provided by squeezing the bag to assist respirations. Bags can be obtained in either rubber or plastic. The rubber deteriorates more rapidly than the plastic, particularly in large cities where atmospheric pollutants are high.

Breathing Tubes and Nasal Masks   The purpose of breathing tubes is to transport the gases from the inhalation sedation unit to the mask or cannula on the patient. Tubes can be made of either corrugated rubber or plastic in a variety of lengths. A selection of connectors should be available to change to different attachments efficiently.

Wide-bore tubes are used to minimize resistance to gas flow. The Magill or Mapelson A circuit is most commonly used in dental inhalation sedation.

The one-way, spring-loaded expiratory valve that permitted escape of exhaled gases with a minimum of pressure has been replaced. We want to prevent the free exit of exhaled gas into the ambient air in an effort to reduce nitrous pollution for office personnel. Scavenging of waste gases is a standard of care in the dental office. The Brown mask, as an example, was designed to incorporate a "mask within a mask." Exhaled gas is expelled into the outer chamber, which is connected to a central suction unit, and the waste gases are removed. Other types of scavenging masks are also available (Fig. 6-20).

The use of a nasal cannula for the delivery of nitrous oxide–oxygen sedation is no longer permissible, because of the excessive flow rates required and the leakage of waste gases that ensues.

The use of an air dilution valve on the nasal hood is not permitted because it cannot be used

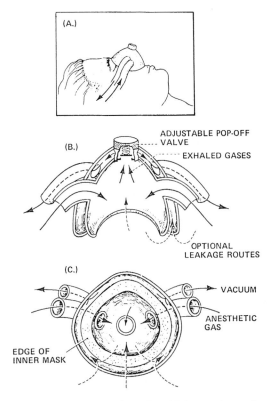

Fig. 6-20. Brown nasal mask, which permits evaluation of exhaled waste gas.

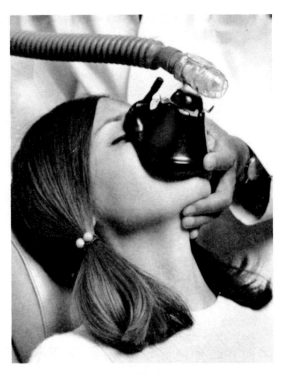

Fig. 6-21. Full face mask should be available to utilize the psychosedation unit as a resuscitator in case of an emergency. Note support of chin and hyperextension of neck to improve airway.

during scavenging. Even so, it was a poor idea, as shown in a study by Hamilton and Eastwood, who inserted a 15-gauge needle into a full face mask. It allowed up to 60% dilution of the inspired gases with room air.[36]

A full face mask (Fig. 6-21) has no place in the nitrous oxide sedation technique but should be available in case of an emergency in which it becomes necessary to provide positive pressure oxygen by squeezing the bag to assist respirations. The nasal mask is easily removed from the breathing tube and the full face mask substituted by means of the appropriate connector.

In regard to the use of 100% oxygen on a patient in distress who continues to deteriorate, it should be a cardinal rule that the use of the machine should be discontinued at least temporarily. Discontinuance gives the operator a chance to observe if the patient improves on room air. If the patient should improve after discontinuance of the 100% "oxygen" from the machine, it would certainly indicate a malfunction of the machine, a rare but possible occurrence.

Cylinders Cylinders come in a variety of sizes, designated A, B, D, E, F, G, H, M, and HH. These cylinders are made of 3/8-inch thick steel and are used to transport and store gases. Interstate Commerce Commission regulations classify any gas with a pressure exceeding 25 psi at 25° C as a compressed gas, and cylinders containing these gases must be subjected to test by interior hydrostatic pressure at least once every 5 years. The Commission requires that the cylinder be marked with the date of the test on the shoulder of the cylinder.

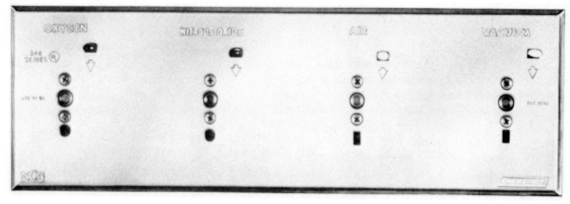

Fig. 6-22.   Coded multiple piping outlet for gases and vacuum.   (Courtesy N.C.G. Division of Chemetron Corp.)

In addition, the American Hospital Association, in cooperation with the American Society of Anesthesiologists and the medical gas industry, has adopted a uniform color code to be used on all gases supplied in standard cylinders:

Oxygen	Green
Nitrous oxide	Light blue
Nitrogen	Gray bottom, orange shoulder
Carbon dioxide	Gray
Cyclopropane	Orange
Helium	Brown
Ethylene	Red

In regard to the ownership of cylinders, sizes A, B, C, and E must be owned by the individual. Cylinder sizes M, G, H, and HH may be owned by the individual, but it is considered economically more feasible to have them supplied by the medical gas supply company. The medical gas industry makes a demurrage charge, per day, on all cylinders (not doctor-owned) that are retained in the office for more than 30 days.

The most frequently used of the smaller cylinders are the E cylinders, which attach directly to the machine. An E cylinder of oxygen contains approximately 625 L. The cost for E cylinders depends on distance from the supplier, number of suppliers in the area, and other variable factors. The E cylinder of nitrous oxide contains approximately 1600 L. Cost can very considerably.

The H cylinder of oxygen and the G cylinder of nitrous oxide are the most frequently used of the larger cylinders and are usually placed in a central storage area. The gases are brought to the piping outlets (Fig. 6-22) from the cylinder storage area through pressure hoses or copper tubing after first passing through a regulator.

The cost of the larger cylinders that are usually not doctor-owned can also vary tremendously, depending on the user's geographic location. An H cylinder of oxygen contains approximately 5300 L. A G cylinder of nitrous oxide contains 13,800 L. Piped gas models from a central supply of large G and H tanks are initially a more expensive installation. They require an initial piping installation, including pressure regulators and gauges, manifold, copper tubing, and wall outlets.

The small cylinder portable models using E size medical gas cylinders require no piping installation. However, the use of the more economical G and H size medical gas cylinders soon offsets the initial expenses.

The handling and storage of cylinders require that:

1. Full cylinders be stored in the vertical position
2. Cylinders be stored in a place of even temperature, particularly avoiding heat
3. Consideration be given to the fact that cylinders should be closed each evening; storage in a place where access is difficult should be avoided

4. Cylinders be handled with care, especially to prevent dropping
5. The use of grease, oil, or other lubricants on the cylinder valve be avoided

In regard to the purity of the gases that are put into these cylinders: it is imperative that these gases be prepared, purified, and filtered according to standards set by the FDA. This can only be ensured through the purchase of the gases from a reputable medical gas supplier.

Instances have been cited in the literature[37,38] of cylinders being contaminated with nitrous dioxide. In the United Kingdom it was discovered that one supplier had distributed 65 cylinders so contaminated. On administration of this contaminated gas, nitric acid was formed, with dire consequences to the patients.

There are two other serious problems that attend the installation of nitrous oxide–oxygen equipment. Isolated incidents have been reported where lines carrying oxygen and nitrous oxide from centralized tanks have been switched during installation. This has resulted in the patient receiving 100% nitrous oxide instead of the intended oxygen. It is important always to check any new installation first, before use, by simply turning on one gas and smelling the outflow. There should be a distinct difference between the odorless oxygen and the characteristic sweetish smell of nitrous oxide. Two severe explosions occurred in dental offices in California with loss of both life and property. The cause was traced to the presence of a Teflon connecting tube and nylon check valve in the oxygen regulator instead of the conventional copper connection. When the oxygen tank was opened, extreme buildup of heat ignited the nylon valve and precipitated these drastic events.[39]

Regulators and Pressure Gauges A reducing valve lowers the stored pressures of the gas in the cylinder to a safe and usable level. The nitrous oxide has a cylinder pressure of 750 psi, and the oxygen has a cylinder pressure of 2400 psi when full. These pressures are reduced by the regulator to an average of 50 to 60 psi in the carrying line.

In regard to the cylinder pressures of the ni-

trous oxide and oxygen, there is a difference in the way the gauges will reflect the depletion of the cylinders. Nitrous oxide is present in the cylinder in a liquified compressed gas and vapor in equilibrium. As long as liquid remains in the cylinder, the gauge shows a cylinder pressure of approximately 750 psi. It is only after the liquid is almost depleted that the pressure begins to drop in relation to the gas outflow. This characteristic makes for an abrupt change from a full cylinder at 750 pounds to an empty cylinder. This characteristic also suggests the need for more than one cylinder of each gas connected to the manifold so that an additional source of the gas is immediately available.

Oxygen is a nonliquified compressed gas, and consequently there is a direct correlation between the pressure recorded on the gauge and the state of depletion of the cylinder.

Manifolds Manifolds can operate automatically, switching from an emptying cylinder to the next full cylinder in the bank. Manifolds can also have an electric audible alarm and signal light that notify the office staff which cylinder is depleted. From these manifolds the gas goes through either high-pressure rubber tubing or copper tubing to wall outlets.

Wall Outlets Wall outlets are supplied by a number of manufacturers. It is important that they too incorporate certain desirable features. These should be quick connectors and have the safety feature of differently spaced and shaped connecting ends. These connectors are coded to fit the proper outlet. From these quick-coupling coded wall connectors should run high-pressure, color-coded hoses to the inhalation sedation unit. The inlets on the machine are fabricated under the Diameter Index Safety System (DISS), which provides threaded connections of a specific diameter to match only a similar diameter connector on the specific hose for each gas. The gas that reaches the machine goes first to the flowmeters.

Safety Measures

It should be office policy to consider the inhalation sedation unit as equipment to be used only for professional purposes: inhalation of ni-

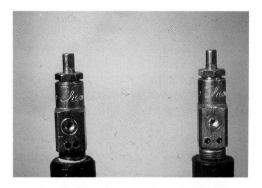

Fig. 6-23. Pin Index Safety System. Note the difference in space between the two holes on the valve surfaces of the nitrous oxide and oxygen cylinders.

trous oxide is not indicated as fun and games for the office staff. In addition, the habit practiced in some offices of a morning "whiff" of the gases to be sure that they are flowing properly is to be discouraged. Nitrous oxide is not addictive, but it can be habit-forming.

All equipment and supplies necessary to perform the planned dental procedures should be immediately available so that the maximal amount of therapy can be performed during the sedation period. The operating team will necessarily be well trained, coordinated, and efficient. The office should have available a sphygmomanometer, a stethoscope, a thermometer, a dental chair that can go into a fully reclining position, and aspirating equipment capable of sucking up at least one-half pint of liquid in 10 seconds.

The inhalation sedation unit may use portable cylinders attached by double yokes. These yokes have an interesting safety feature incorporated into them. There are two pins on the valve surface of the yoke, and there are two holes (Fig. 6-23) drilled in the corresponding surface of the cylinders. Each type of gas has its own combination of pins and holes. This Pin Index Safety System (PISS) makes it almost impossible for the incorrect cylinder of gas to be connected to a yoke that is pin indexed for

another type of gas. The "almost impossibility" of a mismatch was demonstrated by Hogg.[40] He evaluated a newly delivered anesthetic machine and found that the contents of a nitrous oxide cylinder could be delivered through the oxygen yoke and flowmeter and also to the cyclopropane yoke, because of the inexactness of the pin indexing of those particular cylinders. He advised that the system provides only a partial protection and that one must carefully match the color code and cylinder label to the appropriate yoke.

Other desirable features that should be available on all units to enhance the safety and effectiveness of the inhalation sedation equipment are as follows:

1. All gauges and meters should be in full view.
2. The flowmeter scales should be standardized with oxygen on the right.
3. Flowmeters should be calibrated for nitrous oxide and oxygen, with positive control valves controlling the flow. Each complete revolution of the control knob should result in a 1-L increase or decrease in the flow.
4. Flowmeters should be protected and covered with a safety shield.
5. An oxygen monitor should be an integral part of the equipment to verify percent of oxygen coming out of the machine.
6. The push-button oxygen flush should be readily accessible and easily visible on the front of the inhalation sedation unit.
7. All units should have a bag holder tee with a 3- to 5-L bag incorporated into the line. The reservoir bag should be easily observed and resistant to deterioration.
8. The machines should be compact and well made and should incorporate all the previously listed safety features, such as the PISS and DISS systems. The machine should be built to take long hours of use without need for frequent repairs.

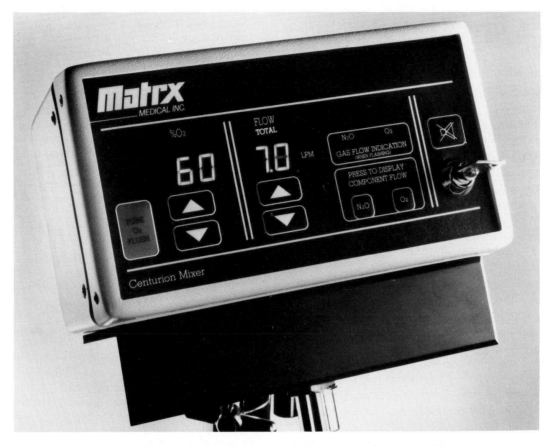

Fig. 6-24. Electronically controlled nitrous oxide and oxygen replacing flowmeters. (Courtesy Matrx Medical Inc.)

9. Electronically monitored flow measurements would provide more accurate control (Fig. 6-24).

Summary

Nitrous oxide–oxygen sedation, properly administered to the conscious child or adult, is an important adjunctive aid to the management of the dental patient. It helps establish enhanced rapport by decreasing anxiety while promoting a more tranquil and often euphoric mood. It cannot be a substitute for local analgesia when painful procedures are undertaken. A minimum concentration of 25% oxygen will ensure adequate oxygenation of the patient. Generally, less than 50% nitrous oxide will suffice to achieve adequate sedation of the patient. Numerous studies have verified the safety of this technique. Our aim is to maintain a conscious and responsive patient free of the hazards of hypoxia and excitement. The desired level of relaxation and sedation is also attainable at much higher levels of oxygenation. Each patient determines his or her own most appropriate concentration of nitrous oxide and oxygen. A stepwise procedure has been presented to facilitate each individual's titration to achieve a baseline of sedation. Concern for the possible harmful effects of trace amounts of nitrous oxide waste prompts the judicious use of lower flow rates, scavenging equipment, and prevention of leaks from defective hoses, attachments, and rubber goods.

Addendum to Chapter 6

Recently a remarkable study relating fertility to nitrous oxide exposure, at high levels, for dental assistants was published.[41] Data were collected from 4850 dental assistants of childbearing age, who worked in offices with and without scavenging as well as other offices where no nitrous oxide was used. Only women who had been pregnant during the past 4 years and worked at least 50 hours per week were included. Other criteria were applied as well, which limited the final group to 459 eligible women.

Within 1 year in this study, 28% of the assistants became pregnant. An increased number of hours of exposure to unscavenged nitrous oxide was significantly associated with decreased fecundability ($P<0.01$). The mean time to conception among women who worked in scavenged offices was similar to that for women working in unexposed offices, while it was much longer for those who worked in unscavenged environments.

The occurrence of spontaneous abortions in 10 pregnant women exposed to high-dose nitrous oxide was 5 out of 10 (50%)! This was compared with an 8% incidence of spontaneous abortion for the other 315 pregnancies in scavenged or non–nitrous oxide offices.

This report provides compelling reasons to use nitrous oxide sedation only under conditions of effective scavenging.

References

1. Dworkin SF et al: Analgesic effects of nitrous oxide with controlled painful stimuli, *J Am Dent Assoc* 107:581-585, 1983.
2. Trieger N et al: Nitrous oxide—a study of physiological and psychological effects, *J Am Dent Assoc* 82(1):142-150 1971.
3. Nitrous oxide–oxygen psychosedation. Report of Council on Dental Therapeutics, *J Am Dent Assoc* 84:393, 1972.
4. Ruben H: Nitrous oxide analgesia for dental patients, *Acta Anaesth Scand (Suppl.* 25:419, 1966.
5. Jaffe M: Nitrous oxide—hemopoietic toxin? *Anesth Prog* 17:8, 1969.
6. Everett FB, Allen CJ: Simultaneous evaluation of cardiorespiratory and analgesic effects of nitrous oxide–oxygen inhalation analgesia, *J Am Dent Assoc* 83:129, 1971.
7. Allen GJ: *Dental anesthesia and analgesia,* ed 3, Baltimore, 1984, Williams & Wilkins.
8. Wynne J et al: Hemodynamic effects of nitrous oxide administered during cardiac catheterization, *J Am Med Assoc* 243(14):1440-1443, 1980.
9. Eisele JH et al: Myocardial performance and N_2O analgesia in coronary artery disease, *Anesthesiology* 44(1):16-20, 1976.
10. Bennett GM et al: Cardiovascular responses to nitrous oxide during enflurane and oxygen anesthesia, *Anesthesiology* 46:227-229, 1977.
11. Philbin DM et al: Nitrous oxide causes myocardial dysfunction, *Anesthesiology* 59(30): A80, 1983.
12. Cohen EN et al: A survey of anesthetic health hazards among dentists, *J Am Dent Assoc* 90:1291-1296, 1975.
13. Whitcher C et al: Development and evaluation of methods for the elimination of waste anesthetic gases and vapors in hospitals. National Institute for Occupational Safety & Health, U.S. Department of Health, Education, and Welfare, May 1975.
14. Kugel G et al: Nitrous oxide and infertility, *Anesth Prog* 37:176, 1990.
15. Nunn JF, Chanarin I. Nitrous oxide inactivates methionine synthetase. In Eger EI, editor: *Nitrous oxide/N$_2$O,* New York, 1985, Elsevier Science Publishing.
16. Layzer RB, Fishman RA, Schafer JA: Neuropathy following abuse of nitrous oxide, *Neurology* 28:505-506, 1978.
17. Sahenk Z et al: Polyneuropathy from inhalation of N_2O cartridges through a whipped cream dispenser, *Neurology* 28:485-487, 1978.
18. Ellis FR et al: Malignant hyperpyrexia induced by nitrous oxide and treated with dexamethasone, *Br Med J* 4:270-271, 1974.
19. Bruce DL, Bach MJ: Psychological studies of human performance as affected by traces of enflurane and nitrous oxide, *Anesthesiology* 42(2):194-196, 1975.
20. National Institute for Occupational Safety and Health: Effects of trace concentrations on anes-

thetic gases on behavioral performance of operating room personnel. National Institute for Occupational Safety and Health, U.S. Department of Health, Education, and Welfare, 1976.

21. Frost EAM: *Central nervous system effects of nitrous oxide.* In Eger EI, editor: *Nitrous oxide N_2O,* New York, 1985, Elsevier Science Publishing.

22. Baden JM: *Mutagencity, carcinogenicity, and teratogenicity of nitrous oxide.* Eger EI, editor: *Nitrous oxide/N_2O,* New York, 1985, Elsevier Science Publishing.

23. Eger EI II, Saidman LJ, Brandstater B: Minimal alveolar anesthetic concentration, *anesthesiology* 26:756, 1965.

24. Hustead RF, Eastwood DW, editors: *Clinical anesthesia:nitrous oxide,* Philadelphia, 1964, FA Davis.

25. Marx GF, Joshi CW, Orkin LR: Placental transmission of nitrous oxide, *Anesthesiology* 32:429, 1970.

26. Smith HT et al: The cardiovascular and sympathomimetic responses to the addition of nitrous oxide to halothane in man, *Anesthesiology* 32:410, 1970.

27. Chapman CR, Murphy TM, Butler SH: Analgesic strength of 33% nitrous oxide: a signal detection theory evaluation, *Science* 179:1246-1248, 1973.

28. Berkowitz BA, Ngai SH, Finck AD: Nitrous oxide "analgesia": resemblance to opiate action, *Science* 194:967-968.

29. Finck AD: *Nitrous oxide analgesia.* In EI Eger, editor: *Nitrous oxide/N_2O,* New York, 1985, Elsevier Science Publishing.

30. Chen DC, Quock RM: A study of central opioid involvement in nitrous oxide analgesia in mice, *Anesth Prog* 37:181, 1990.

31. Bender L: *A visual motor Gestalt test and its clinical use,* New York, 1983, American Orthopsychiatric Association.

32. Duncan GH, Moore P: Nitrous oxide and the dental patient: a review of adverse reactions, *J Am Dent Assoc* 108:213-219, 1984.

33. Jastak JT, Malamed SF: Nitrous oxide sedation and sexual phenomena, *J Am Dent Assoc* 101:38-40, 1980.

34. McCarthy FM, Shuken RA: Appraisal of the demand flow anesthetic machine and review of the literature, *J Oral Surg* 27:624, 1969.

35. Allen GD, Gehrig JD, Tolas AC: An evaluation of demand-flow anesthetic machines in dental practice, *J Am Dent Assoc* 78:91, 1969.

36. Hamilton WK, Eastwood DW: A study of denitrogenation with some inhalation anesthetic systems, *Anesthesiology* 16:861, 1955.

37. Albright RL, Bakett JA: Poisonous effects of the impurities of nitrous oxide, *J Oral Surg* 26:643, 1968.

38. Higher oxides of nitrogen as an impurity of nitrous oxide (editorial), *Br J Anaesth* 39(5):343-344, 1967.

39. Follmar KE: Anesthetic gas fires are preventable, *Anesth Prog* 19:2, 1972.

40. Hogg CE: Pin-indexing failures, *Anesthesiology* 38(1):85-86, 1973.

41. Rowland AS, Baird DD, Weinberg CR, Shore DL, Shy CM, Wilcox AJ: Reduced fertility among women employed as dental assistants exposed to high levels of nitrous oxide, *N Eng J Med* 324:14, 993-997, 1992.

7

Intravenous Sedation

"I don't mind a needle anywhere else but in my mouth, Doctor." This and other similar comments often made by dental patients amplify the neurologic and psychologic sensitivity of the oral cavity. The mouth and face are richly innervated and also heavily invested with emotional significance. Although avoidance of regular dental care is often attributed to economic limitations, removal of these financial concerns usually exposes them as mere rationalizations for the patient's more basic fear and anxiety. Dentists have become increasingly aware of the need for "something" to influence the psyche of the patient while the local anesthetic blocks the pain. The old punitive "sit still and take it" attitude is fortunately fast fading from the practitioner's routine.

A variety of helpful approaches to patient management are presented in this book. No one method is a panacea. Although office general anesthesia has been developed to a high degree primarily by oral surgeons who have had advanced education and training in its use, they constitute a small percentage of practicing dentists and are obviously limited by their specialization to surgical procedures. An even smaller number of general dentists have taken graduate anesthesia training, of at least 1 year's duration, and can provide more comprehensive dental care.

Sections of this chapter are reprinted from Trieger N: Intravenous sedation: symposium on anesthesia and analgesia, *Dent Clin North Am* 17:2, 249-261 April 1973; and Trieger N: Emergencies and complications from sedation modalities, *Dent Clin North Am* 17:3, 429-442 July 1973.

For most dentists and patients, dentistry under general anesthesia would be ill advised and unnecessary. Nevertheless, "something"[1] is needed to enhance patient acceptance of dental treatment. Nitrous oxide–oxygen psychosedation (see Chapter 6) has been widely accepted as a helpful modality for managing the conscious dental patient.

Expanding the doctor's scope of patient management has also included the use of oral and intramuscular premedication. Both these routes are subject to considerable variation in patient response, take longer to exert their effect and to wear off, and require, at best, an approximation of the appropriate dosage. The most reliable way to achieve the desired effect of a drug is to titrate it slowly, directly into the bloodstream, anticipating objective and subjective signs and symptoms in the conscious, responding patient.

The ultimate aim of intravenous sedation is to achieve a level of relaxation and cooperation without obtundation and compromise of vital functions. It must be emphasized that there is no predetermined dosage and that each patient must be individually titrated to his or her own effect. The smallest dose administered that achieves relaxation and cooperation is the proper dose for that patient. Local anesthesia must be administered for any anticipated painful procedures. It will be more profound in its effect because of the control of the patient's anxiety by the intravenous agent.

Patient Selection

"How dare we inject anything into a patient without first ascertaining that individual's medical history and recording vital signs such as

blood pressure, pulse, and respiratory rate.'' Dr. Seymour Carr of Los Angeles would regularly and dramatically challenge his students with this remark—even when discussing the use of local anesthesia. This point is well taken, especially when one considers the administration of potent agents that can affect primary physiologic functions.

Each patient must be queried in depth to ascertain present state of health, past medical history, any specific medications being taken, and allergies or adverse drug reactions. Baseline, pretreatment records should include notation of the vital signs. Medical consultation should be sought when indicated. Those dentists with limited experience would do well to select Class I and II risk patients—healthy individuals without history or evidence of complicating medical illnesses.

During the pretreatment visit it is wise to look specifically for the presence of easily accessible veins, either on the dorsum of the hands or in the antecubital fossae. The absence of readily visible or palpable superficial veins may influence you in patient selection. The more experienced operator will ''find'' veins that the anatomy books had overlooked. By carefully checking for available veins before scheduling a session under intravenous sedation, the operator will avoid the unnecessary trauma of multiple punctures.

Technique Selection

The technique strongly advocated is one that utilizes a continuous intravenous drip attached to an indwelling, short 21-gauge needle (Fig. 7-1). This setup is preferable to the ''hit-and-run technique'' of intravenous injection. It offers a number of decided advantages as well as a few disadvantages. Primarily, it ensures a safe, patent line into the vein. Before injecting any drug, one can readily (and repeatedly) make sure that the needle is properly positioned and that it is neither outside the vein nor in a superficial artery (Figs. 7-2 and 7-3). The saline reservoir bag also serves to flush the line should any reaction develop or dilution be desired. It also maintains an open line so that additional medication may be given as needed through a

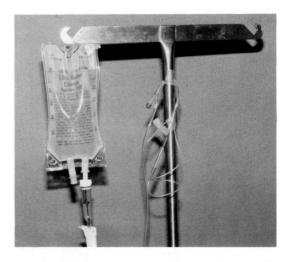

Fig. 7-1. Once the intravenous line has been established, it is maintained with a slow infusion of saline or dextrose/water.

small rubber diaphragm in the tubing assembly, whether to prolong the treatment period or in the event of emergency to administer other agents (Fig. 7-4).

The short 21-gauge scalp vein needle (e.g., Abbott-Butterfly) is well beveled, not readily dislodged, and easily secured by clear tape (Fig. 7-5). This size will permit at least 13 ml/min to flow through the system, compared to a smaller 23-gauge needle, which only allows only 3 ml/min to pass in. The tape should be applied so that portion of the butterfly wing nearest the tubing is left uncovered. This serves two purposes: (1) it helps to keep the needle pointed downward into the lumen of the vein and avoid contact with the vein wall, and (2) subsequent removal of the tape will not disturb the needle and further traumatize the vein if the needle can be stabilized by the operator's finger while the tape is being removed.

Objections to the regular use of this technique of continuous intravenous drip include the somewhat higher cost for the intravenous (IV) fluids, tubing, and needle and the view that ''hanging up a bag in the dental office may make it appear like a hospital.'' This latter remark often reflects the apprehension and inexperience of the operator. Patients generally ac-

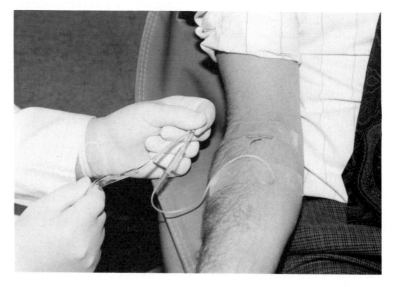

Fig. 7-2. Pinching the venotube prior to the injection of any drug helps to ensure that the needle is within the vein.

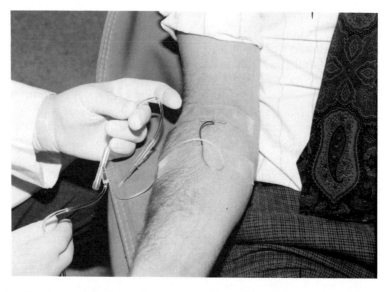

Fig. 7-3. Releasing the obstruction of the tube causes a reflux of blood into the capillary tube, verifying the correct location of a patent needle.

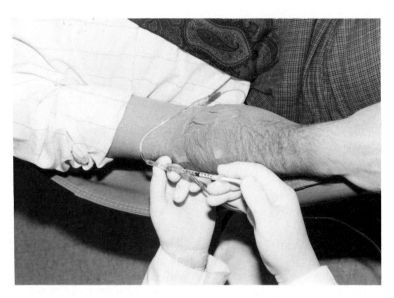

Fig. 7-4. Subsequent drug administration is done slowly by individual titration for objective and subjective effects.

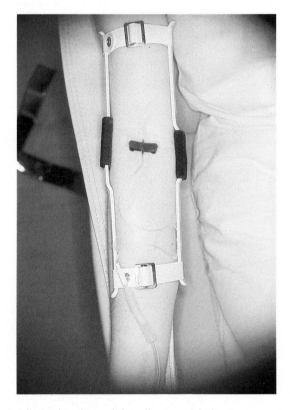

Fig. 7-5. Additional restraint limits bending of the elbow and helps to prevent dislodging of the needle. Lemco splint (Littell's Oxygen, Inc., North Hollywood, Calif.) is being used. Needle is readily visualized through clear tape, which helps to prevent extravascular infusion.

cept dentists' methods and materials if these are incorporated into the routine. IV bags are best suspended behind the patient rather than in full view, so that the apprehensive patient does not become alarmed by intently watching a harmless bubble floating down the tubing.

The tourniquet is applied snugly and the arm is suspended dependently. The patient is requested to "pump" by opening and closing the fist. Allow ample time for veins to fill. Hecker, Lewis, and Stanley[2] have shown that rubbing a small amount of nitroglycerin ointment between the fingers or over the metacarpal area 2 hours before significantly enhanced the venipuncture, when compared with a placebo group or the untreated hand.

The skin is prepped with alcohol and the venipuncture is made by directing the needle, bevel up, at an angle of about 30 degrees to the surface of the skin (Fig. 7-6). With one motion, the skin and vessel wall are pierced. The angle of the needle is decreased, and the needle is threaded up into the lumen of the vein. Blood immediately appears in the capillary tubing at-tached to the needle. The tourniquet is released, the IV tubing clamp is opened, and saline is allowed to run into the vein. The needle is secured with clear tape. If the veins are large, the dorsum of the hand is a preferred site for venipuncture, especially if the operator tenses the overlying skin and the patient closes his or her fingers over the operator's two fingers. The primary preferred site is the lateral aspect of the antecubital fossa. Here the vessels are generally larger but may be less apparent, especially in female patients (Fig. 7-7).

The medial aspect of the antecubital fossa may also show prominent veins, but in a small percentage of patients a superficial branch of the brachial artery may be present. It is wise to palpate this area for arterial pulsations prior to placing the tourniquet. If the antecubital fossa is used, an arm board or splint will be required to prevent the patient from flexing the arm and dislodging the needle. Once this setup is secured and the IV is running, the appropriate drug may be drawn up in a syringe for administration into the tubing diaphragm (Fig. 7-8).

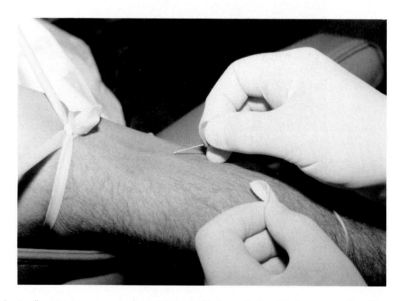

Fig. 7-6.   The butterfly wings are grasped, and the needle is angled at 30 degrees to the skin surface. Skin and vein are pierced in one motion; then the angle is decreased and the needle is threaded up the vein's lumen.

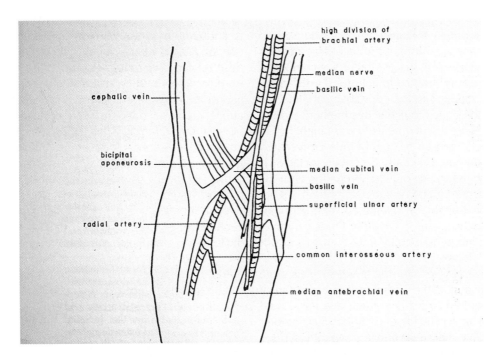

Fig. 7-7. Anatomic schema of the antecubital fossa, showing locations of major medial and lateral veins and communicating vein. The superficial location of a branch of the brachial artery on the medial aspect invites caution so as to avoid an intra-arterial puncture.

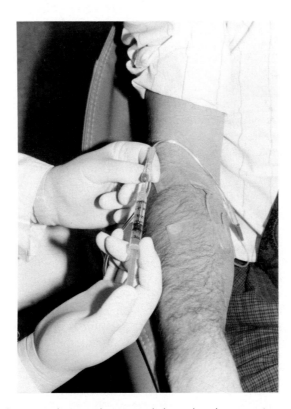

Fig. 7-8. Increments of diazepam being administered through a larger syringe with the intravenous line flowing rapidly to minimize burning sensation.

Drug Selection

The Jorgensen Technique A large number of agents have been used for intravenous sedation techniques in dentistry. Various combinations of drugs are administered to achieve a satisfactory level of sedation in the conscious patient. One of the oldest and more effective methods, which has stood the test of time well, was taught by Dr. Neils B. Jorgensen of Loma Linda University.[3] The technique, originally described in 1953, is designed to provide only light sedation with the use of pentobarbital sodium (Nembutal), meperidine hydrochloride (Demerol), and scopolamine. Each patient is carefully titrated intravenously with pentobarbital until the first signs of cortical depression are elicited—slight drowsiness, dizziness, or blurring of vision. This stage is designated as the "baseline." The amount of drug required to achieve this stage has varied from 30 mg to 300 mg of pentobarbital sodium. Meperidine then is given via a separate syringe according to a dosage schedule related to the barbiturate already administered: that is, 25 mg of meperidine hydrochloride per 100 mg of pentobarbital sodium; or 12.5 mg of meperidine hydrochloride per 50 mg of pentobarbital sodium. The arbitrary *maximum* dose for this technique is 25 mg of meperidine hydrochloride. Scopolamine hydrobromide 0.32 mg is given together with the meperidine.

For hypertensive or elderly patients only baseline is reached and very little, if any, of the meperidine is used. Extreme caution is advised for hypertensive patients who are already receiving antihypertensive medications.

The value of barbiturate premedication has been demonstrated both to effect sedation and to protect against local anesthetic toxicity.[4,5] In a well-designed study of the Jorgensen technique, Everett and Allen found no significant changes in arterial blood pressure, central venous pressure, cardiac output, total peripheral resistance, Pao_2, or $Paco_2$.[6] The cardiac rate showed a progressive decrease, with the exception of a transient increase immediately after nerve block. The results of this study confirm that there is minimal physiologic upset associated with this technique, although 3 of the 10

subjects studied developed nausea. This nausea is attributable to the narcotic and constitutes one of the drawbacks of this technique; it is dose related. Narcotics also block the reflexes from receptors in the carotid sinus, aortic arch, and pulmonary vessels, permitting wide fluctuations in blood pressure with orthostatic hypotension developing when the patient assumes an erect position.[7] Intravenous meperidine, given rapidly or in higher dosage, is known to cause significant decreases in respiratory rate, minute volume, and arterial oxygen tension, with an increase in $Paco_2$ and a decrease in the ventilatory response to carbon dioxide—all indicative of significant respiratory depression even at blood concentrations less than those required for analgesia.[8]

Other adverse reactions include flushing, sweating, weakness, and tachycardia. In some patients meperidine triggers a histamine release[9]; locally, this may appear as discrete erythema involving the superficial veins of the forearm receiving the intravenous infusion (Fig. 7-9).

Pentobarbital, in some patients, has the tendency to produce prolonged drowsiness, lethargy, and residual sedation ("hangover"). Studies of recovery from intravenous sedation with both Nembutal and Demerol showed a mean of 85 minutes, almost 50% longer than with other agents used in this study.[10] Caution is advised in the use of sedatives and narcotics in patients receiving antidepressant drugs, particularly the monoamine oxidase (MAO) inhibitors: Marplan, Nardil, and Parnate are three examples of MAO inhibitors used primarily as antidepressants that can interact dangerously with strong analgesics and produce severe depressant effects.

The anticholinergic agents, such as atropine and scopolamine, used to reduce salivary secretions and, in the case of scopolamine, to enhance a dissociative psychic effect, must be used with caution in patients with tachycardia. Occasionally, larger doses of intravenous atropine (0.8 to 1.0 mg), especially in patients with ischemic heart disease, may precipitate adverse ventricular arrhythmias. Doses as small as 0.2

and 0.3 mg are reported to produce increased vagal tone leading to further bradycardia.[11] Contrary to popular belief, the usual doses used do not increase intraocular pressure even in patients with glaucoma.[12] Scopolamine may also cause disorientation in the elderly patient and in the very young patient.

Dentistry has played a primary role in the quest for more satisfactory sedative agents for ambulatory care. Unlike the hospitalized surgical patient who is premedicated, wheeled to the operating room, anesthetized, and then returned to a supervised recovery room, the office dental patient poses a different kind of management problem. The patient for sedation in the office must be rendered relaxed and cooperative in a short period of time, receive local anesthesia to block peripheral pain, and be able to walk out of the office and travel home in the company of a responsible adult. These requirements have prompted dentists to develop intravenous techniques utilizing other agents.

The Shane Technique Dr. Sylvan Shane of Baltimore, Maryland, taught the use of a combination of an intravenous narcotic such as alphaprodine hydrochloride (Nisentil), hydroxyzine hydrochloride (Vistaril, Atarax), atropine, and methohexital sodium (Brevital) plus local anesthesia and considerable verbal conditioning by the operator.[13] This technique has many enthusiastic advocates but has several limitations. Hydroxyzine is no longer recommended for intravenous use by its manufacturers. The combination of a potent narcotic, sedative, and hypnotic such as methohexital often produces a patient who verges on general anesthesia. Any technique that uses methohexital requires the knowledge, skill, and equipment to manage the fully anesthetized, unconscious patient. This has been commonly regarded, in the United States, as the province of those who have had at least a year of advanced education and training in general anesthesia. Both thiopental sodium (Pentothal) and methohexital are potent hypnotics with narrow dosage margins between unconsciousness and consciousness and cannot be recommended for use as a conscious technique of light sedation.[14]

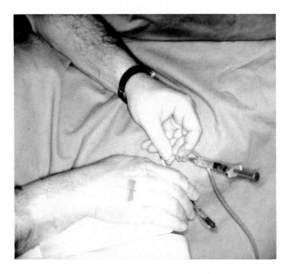

Fig. 7-9. Although smaller veins on the dorsum of the hand are readily accessible, burning on drug administration is more prevalent.

Dr. Shane has recently modified his technique by significantly reducing the dosages administered. For example, children receive only 25 mg hydroxyzine hydrochloride, no more than 6 mg alphaprodine hydrochloride, and no more than 5 mg methohexital sodium. Adults are given 50 mg hydroxyzine hydrochloride, 24 mg alphaprodine hydrochloride, and 5 mg methohexital sodium. All patients receive local anesthesia. He does not advocate the use of adjunctive oxygen or nitrous oxide.

Other agents such as secobarbital sodium (Seconal) and promethazine hydrochloride (Phenergan) have been used in combination with narcotics to effect sedation. Promethazine is a phenothiazine and shows marked potentiating effects when used with other depressants. It also has a long-lasting action and produces adrenergic blocking effects that can cause vasodilatation and hypotension, resistant to reversal by vasopressors.

Diazepam (Valium) Clinically, intravenous sedation with diazepam is qualitatively different from that with pentobarbital. Diazepam produces less drowsiness than pentobarbital and more signs of relaxation. Anxiety-reducing properties of drugs are said to be mediated by the cyclic AMP system in the brain. Diazepam is a potent inhibitor of cyclic AMP activity. Data indicate that there is a relationship between the effect of a drug on conflict behavior and its ability to inhibit cyclic AMP phosphodiesterase activity in the brain.[15] In this same study, pentobarbital did not inhibit the activity of cyclic AMP phosphodiesterase.

Drugs described as serotonin antagonists also produce anxiety reduction similar to the effects of the benzodiazepines (diazepam) and barbiturates: they decrease the turnover of norepinephrine, serotonin, and other biogenic amines in the brain. This effect may be responsible for some of the behavioral responses of tranquilizers.[16]

Diazepam has demonstrated effective control of seizures in both humans and animals.[17,18] The primary sites of action of diazepam are said to be the limbic system and those subcortical areas of the brain that are concerned with emotions, that is, the midbrain, reticular formation, hypothalamus, and thalamus. Various studies indicate that diazepam blocks pressor responses by central, supraspinal mechanisms rather than peripheral mechanisms, with a major locus of depressant action on the brainstem reticular system.[19]

Further developments in the field of neuropharmacology have focused on the influence of various neurotransmitters and receptors. Glycine and gamma-aminobutyric acid (GABA) are endogenous substances that inhibit neurotransmission at specific receptor sites. The benzodiazepines enhance the affinity of these neuromodulators for their receptors. The benzodiazepine receptor sites, although not identical, are located very near glycine and GABA binding sites. Recent work has identified a related imidazobenzepine that specifically blocks the binding sites of diazepam without producing any other pharmacologic effects. This drug, RO 15-1778, available now as flumazenil (Mazicon), is highly effective in specifically reversing the effects of benzodiazepines.[20]

Giving diazepam intravenously requires a slow infusion of not more than 5 mg (1 ml)/min. It is recommended by the manufacturer that diazepam not be mixed or diluted with other drugs or solutions. However, injecting this agent into a running saline infusion has been found to significantly diminish the burning sensation usually experienced and to have no adverse effect on the dosage or reaction to the drug. When contacting the saline, a whitish, flocculent precipitate forms that readily resuspends in the bloodstream.[21] In general, experience has shown that most young adults will tolerate 10 mg to 20 mg diazepam injected slowly to achieve a level of lessened anxiety. Consistently, older patients are remarkably susceptible to very small doses of intravenous diazepam, individual titration of 2 to 5 mg will be found adequate to sedate them.

Dalen et al evaluated the hemodynamic and respiratory effects of diazepam during cardiac catheterization when 5 to 10 mg was given intravenously.[22] One half of the patients showed slight blood pressure decrease with no significant changes occurring in heart rate, stroke volume, pulmonary artery pressure, or peripheral resistance. Hypoventilation occurred in all patients, but these changes were without clinical correlates and required no specific treatment.

In a study by Gross, Smith, and Smith measuring ventilatory response to carbon dioxide after intravenous diazepam in high dosage (0.4 mg/kg), ventilatory depression began within 1 minute and persisted for 25 minutes.[23] They concluded that diazepam in large doses was capable of producing respiratory depression but in combination with narcotics or other central nervous system (CNS) depressants there are further additive or synergistic effects even at lower dose levels. Large doses of the narcotic antagonist naloxone hydrochloride have been shown to reverse some of the ventilatory depression induced by diazepam.[24]

Driscoll et al, using intravenous diazepam in doses of up to 30 mg, found no single sign or symptom to be reliably indicative of the level of depression.[25] They reported a level of amnesia for the local anesthetic injection of 54% on the day of surgery and 70% at the postoperative visit. Amnesia is usually greater for those events occurring shortly after the diazepam is given and becomes more manifest when the patient is questioned after several days. O'Neill et al found that the administration of 0.3 mg/kg of diazepam produced amnesia in almost 80% of their patients.[26] Interestingly, they advise, "Diazepam is most effective when used for an operation which in unapprehensive patients would be considered feasible under local anesthesia in daily practice."

Healy, Edmondson, and Dudley Hall reported its use in mentally handicapped patients: males over 15 years of age required 25 mg and females 20 mg.[27] Children between the ages of 10 to 15 years required 10 mg on the average. Hyperactive retarded children may require higher doses; however, the use of general anesthesia is often preferable.

Gregg, Ryan, and Levin found the amnesic action of diazepam to be better than nitrous oxide, meperidine, or scopolamine.[28] Anterograde amnesia and duration were both related to dosage and applied equally to visual, auditory, and painful events. The peak of the amnesic effect was 2 to 10 minutes at lower doses, whereas a dose of 30 mg (approximately one half the dose needed for general anesthesia) produced 100% amnesia for longer periods. The main amnesic effect appeared to be the result of interference with consolidation of long-term memory. Gelfman et al agreed with Gregg that the acquisition phase of learning and memory were not affected by sedation but that consolidation into long-term memory was impaired.[29]

Kaufman et al suggest that the amnesic and anxiolytic properties of diazepam may also serve to modulate pain, although the drug has no direct analgesic properties.[30]

Healy and Vickers reported their study of laryngeal competence under diazepam using 0.2 mg/kg.[31] Radiographically opaque medium placed on the tongue was discernible on a chest radiograph shortly after administration of IV diazepam in 8 of 19 patients tested (42%). These authors concluded that the cough reflex did not provide adequate protection against aspiration.

Although diazepam has been found effective as the sole sedative agent (plus local anesthesia) for most patients, there are those who insist on being totally unconscious. It is an abuse of conscious sedation technique to push any drug to unsafe limits if the patient is really best managed under a general anesthetic. All our efforts should go toward providing a safe, comfortable, and more cooperative patient who understands that he or she will *not* be asleep but will also not be acutely and anxiously aware of the dental treatment.

Various agents have been used, in combination, to help produce a better conscious sedative effect and gain the patient's cooperation. Multiple drugs usually result in a deeper level of sedation and a greater incidence of untoward side effects.

Intravenous Procedure with Diazepam With the intravenous line opened to full flow, a test dose of 2.0 to 2.5 mg is administered to each patient and 2 to 3 minutes allowed to note the reaction. Elderly patients should receive a 1-mg test dose. Although a cloudy white suspension is seen at the interface of the drug and the saline in the line, this has not been found to influence the drug's effect clinically. The administration then continues slowly, and the operator should look for specific objective, but often subtle, signs of light sedation.

For example, the hands gripping the arm rests may relax; the patient's posture may change from tension to ease; the legs, extended horizontally, may splay and the shoe tips point outward. All the while, the operator stays in verbal contact with the patient, who reports feeling "lightheaded" or more relaxed and less "uptight." The British practice of giving diazepam until ptosis occurs (Verrill sign)[26,32,33] produces a sedation that is often deeper than necessary. In reporting his studies on the use of diazepam for general anesthesia, Dr. Verrill noted a drooping

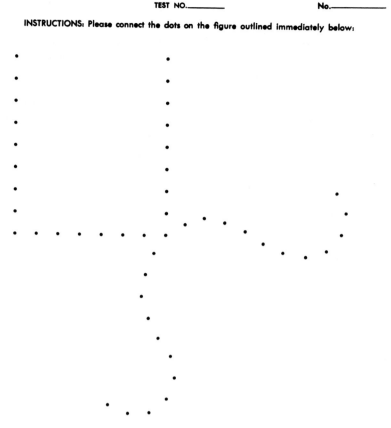

TEST NO._____   No._____

INSTRUCTIONS: Please connect the dots on the figure outlined immediately below:

Fig. 7-10. Modified Bender Motor Gestalt Test, used for studies of drug effect and recovery of psychomotor performance.

of the eyelids when his patients were going progressively deeper under sedation. Dr. Drummond-Jackson is said to have interrupted Dr. Verrill's presentation to exclaim that "at last—now a sign had been found to use for diazepam sedation and henceforth, we shall call it the 'Verrill sign'." It must be understood that this sign represents a significant level of CNS depression with attendant respiratory depression and, for most patients undergoing conscious sedation, is unwarranted. In addition to the subtle postural and conversational changes already noted, the lightly sedated patient may show some slurring of speech, become loquacious, and ask the same question several times despite receiving an appropriate answer. Diazepam, unlike nitrous oxide, does not produce a "high" or a euphoric state. It just removes the heightened level of awareness and exaggerated responses to stress. When the titration has been achieved, the intravenous line is slowed to one drop every 8 to 10 seconds just to maintain an open line and avoid clotting the needle.

Driscoll's ECG tracings revealed a high incidence of minor cardiac dysrhythmias during local anesthesia and surgery (21% of the younger patients); a similar percentage experienced dysrhythmias during the second procedure under sedation. Under local anesthesia alone, almost 46% of the older patients experienced dysrhythmias, whereas under sedation 29% showed abnormalities.[25] In our experience as well, light intravenous sedation tempers the stress of the dental appointment and is reflected in a lesser incidence of dysrhythmias induced by endogenous catecholamines.

Table 7-1 Average dosages for all drugs

GROUP	DRUG	AVERAGE DOSE
I Local (control)	Lidocaine hydrochloride	2.5 ml
II Meperidine	Meperidine hydrochloride	79.3 mg
III Diazepam	Diazepam	10.5 mg
	Meperidine hydrochloride	54.5 mg
IV Hydroxyzine	Hydroxyzine hydrochloride	52.8 mg
	Meperidine hydrochloride	63.9 mg
V Pentobarbital	Pentobarbital sodium	56.9 mg
	Meperidine hydrochloride	69.4 mg
VI Methohexital (control)	Methohexital sodium	132.2 mg
	Meperdine hydrochloride	38.2 mg
	Hydroxyzine hydrochloride	53.5 mg

Table 7-2 Psychomotor effects of drugs

DRUG GROUP	PERFORMANCE
Local control (I) and meperidine (II) only	No significant effect
Diazepam and meperidine (III) and hydroxyzine and meperidine (IV)	Minor effect
Pentobarbital and meperidine (V)	Moderate effect
General anesthesia control of methohexital	Profound impairment

Recovery

Rapid recovery from sedation is essential to successful ambulatory care of dental patients. Clinical approximations of recovery are very variable and subject to operator as well as patient bias. Nonobjective studies of recovery from intravenous diazepam show wide variations, from 20 minutes to 90 minutes.[26,32,36] To provide more objective criteria of drug effect and recovery, a simple drawing test was developed with the aid of one of the basic figures from the Bender Motor Gestalt test series.[34,35] This test requires the patient to simply connect the dots of the diagram provided (Fig. 7-10). It enables each patient to provide his or her own starting baseline; the test is then repeated at subsequent intervals. The results of the test may be easily scored numerically as "number of dots missed." As recovery ensues, psychomotor performance improves and the original baseline score is achieved.[35] Objective scoring shows that return to the patient's own psychomotor baseline was almost complete in 60 minutes after diazepam was administered, whereas older patients required 90 minutes.[25,36,37] Nembutal/Demerol recoveries required longer than 85 minutes even in younger patients.

Our comparative study[36] of several commonly used sedative agents included both local anesthetic and general anesthetic control groups. Results from this report are shown in Tables 7-1 and 7-2.

Vital signs showed no significant drug-related differences. All measurements fell within a normal tolerance range. Dalen et al[22] also reported that systemic blood pressure and heart rate did not change significantly following intravenous administration of diazepam in similar doses (5

Table 7-3 Recovery times of various drugs

DRUG GROUP	RECOVERY TIME (MIN)
Local anesthesia (control I) and meperidine only (control II)	<5
Diazepam and meperidine	60
Hydroxyzine and meperidine	75
Pentobarbital and meperidine	85
Methohexital, hydroxyzine, and meperidine	80

to 10 mg). However, they did note a significant reduction in ventilation, due primarily to decreases in tidal volume.

Table 7-3 indicates the recovery times obtained with the various agents studied.

With the technique of a continuously open IV, one can add increments of sedative drugs as the procedure requires, taking advantage of the knowledge of recovery time. Although psychomotor recovery is complete after 1 to 1 ½ hours, the drug is by no means all dissipated by that time. It is being deconjugated and excreted over the next several hours and days. Baird and Hailey have shown that diazepam serum levels decrease radidly but then show a rise with recurrence of drowsiness approximately 6 hours after administration of the drugs.[37]

Patients should be allowed to recover in the office and then be taken home afterward. They should be advised to refrain from drinking any alcoholic beverages and cautioned about the potential for enhanced depressant effects of other CNS drugs. It is also wise to suggest that the patient defer making complicated or fine judgments for the remainder of that day. Good experiences of tranquility and subsequent restful naps, without "hangovers", are common following such dental treatment sessions.

The "Trieger Dot Test" has been used by others in a number of studies to evaluate psychomotor effects of drugs and recovery. It is a simple, inexpensive, paper-and-pencil test that does not involve any special apparatus and is not influenced by learning. Letourneau and Denis evaluated the test and reported its reliability and validity.[38]

Complications of Intravenous Sedation

Complications may be considered in several different categories: (1) complications of venipuncture technique; (2) complications of adverse drug reactions and interactions; (3) complications secondary to underlying medical illness.

VENIPUNCTURE TECHNIQUE

Hematoma Formation The commonest complication is the formation of a hematoma. Leakage of blood into the interstitial tissue leads to localized swelling and discoloration. The needle itself, properly placed, acts to obturate this minute opening and prevent leakage. Immediately after the needle is removed, pressure is applied to the injection site to prevent extravasation of blood. Localized hematomas are best treated with direct pressure and subsequent application of hot packs to the area.

Infiltration Outside the Vein Infiltration outside the vein may also occur if the technique is poor or the needle becomes dislodged. One of the primary advantages of the short "butterfly" needle is the ease with which it can be secured with clear tape to prevent displacement. Should infiltration occur with the technique recommended in this chapter, only saline will be administered. This solution is isotonic and is very rapidly absorbed without tissue injury. No drug should ever be injected until the operator confirms the needle's location to be within the vein. This is readily done by squeezing the IV tubing and releasing it to see a short column of blood flow back up into the capillary tubing of the "butterfly" assembly (see Figs. 7-2 and 7-3).

This patent needle will now ensure a rapid flow of saline from the reservoir bag and provide a safe conduit for drug administration. It is also advisable to avoid covering up the IV site with the drape or bib. Should infiltration develop, it can be readily noticed by swelling in the area and by the slowing of the rate of drip despite opening the stopcock.

The use of a needle catheter (Angiocath) may be helpful as a substitute for the butterfly. It is less likely to become dislodged when the patient moves; however, it is more expensive and requires additional assistance when it is being connected to the intravenous assembly.

Venospasm Occasionally, a patient experiences a burning sensation in the area of the venipuncture even in the absence of drug instillation. This is probably due to the spasm secondary to the trauma of needle insertion and soon fades.

A burning sensation is also commonly produced in patients receiving diazepam. They should be alerted to this possiblity and advised that it will fade, especially if the saline drip is opened wide to flush the vein. Meperidine occasionally produces a release of histamine, and the superficial vessels of the forearm or upper arm will glow like an infrared photograph. Flushing with saline will also resolve this reaction within a few minutes.

Phlebothrombosis Unlike the thrombophlebitis that develops in a fair percentage of hospitalized patients receiving various IV fluids over several days, phlebothrombosis is more benign. Unless the original needle and equipment are contaminated, in which case a true thrombophlebitis may develop, the infrequent occurrence of the phlebothrombosis secondary to a short IV sedation session is probably related to localized trauma by the needle or the drug. It tends to occur in patients with a prior history of other episodes of venous thrombosis and may represent an individual susceptibility—not necessarily limited to any particular age or sex. Fortunately, this firm, tender, localized swelling is usually without other evidence of inflammation and responds readily to hot packs. Although embolization occasionally occurs from thromboses of the deep leg veins and pelvic veins, this does not appear to be the case with thromboses of hand and arm veins with the technique advocated. Hoare reported a case of a pulmonary embolus secondary to diazepam injected into an antecubital vein for an endoscopic procedure in a 47-year-old man. Phlebograms of the lower extremities failed to show any thrombi. A large (5-cm) thrombus was demonstrated at the original venipuncutre site.[39]

Patients experienceing a burning sensation on administration of diazepam are more likely to develop a localized phlebothrombosis.[40] This occurs more often when the vein is small or the titration is done rapidly. A slow administration into a large vessel with the intravenous solution flowing full open will minimize the burning and the incidence of phlebothrombosis. The vehicle carrying diazepam is propylene glycol, which is very irritating to the vein wall, especially in concentration. Gelfman, Dionne, and Driscoll demonstrated a significantly higher incidence of phlebothrombosis when hand veins were used.[40] Neither smoking nor oral contraceptives influenced the incidence of phlebothrombosis. Treatment usually involves the application of hot packs to the area and anti-inflammatory analgesics as needed. Anticoagulant medications are generally not indicated. With the passage of time, the thrombus is absorbed and the vein regains patency.

Intra-Arterial Injections By palpating for pulsations prior to placing the tourniquet, by being wary especially of the medial aspect of the antecubital fossa, and by using the IV technique recommended in this chapter, intra-arterial injections can be avoided. If the needle does strike an artery, there is usually greater discomfort; blood will rise very rapidly into the tubing and may be seen to pulsate. The IV drip will cease or slow dramatically. Pain *peripheral* to the site of injections of drug into arteries has been reported to herald severe tissue damage and gangrene of the fingers.[41]

Therapy is aimed at preventing thrombosis of the artery and its resultant ischemic tissue changes. Heparinization to minimize clotting is recommended, and supportive measures such as adequate hydration and pain medications are given. Sympathetic ganglion nerve blocks have been de-emphasized, although they may help to diminish further reflex vasoconstriction in response to pain. Intra-arterial procaine has not been found to be helpful.[42] Blockage of a medium-sized artery may be amenable to early vascular bypass surgery or to the early use of one of the new clot-dissolving enzymes such as streptokinase or urokinase.

DRUG REACTIONS AND INTERACTIONS

Hypersensitivity Hypersensitivity reactions may occur with any drug. A careful history prior to treatment is mandatory. Acute anaphylactoid reactions constitute an immediate threat to life. The availability of an open IV line, as recommended, would greatly facilitate emergency care. Details of the management of such acute reactions are discussed in Chapter 9.

Drug Overdose Overdose should never occur with the technique of light sedation advocated here. There is no need to administer an arbitrary dosage—in fact, this technique is the most accurate way to provide medication by individual titration. With the availability of an open IV line, the operator can always give more drug, if necessary, without having to repuncture the patient. One should be familiar with the signs and symptoms of light sedation and work within this framework.

Individual variability of reaction is represented in the composite by the bell-shaped curve of distribution. Some patients will be extraordinarily sensitive to small doses of drug, some will be remarkably resistant, but most of the population will respond somewhere in between. Inadvertent overdosage with depression of respiration and other vital functions dictates the need to support ventilation and, if necessary, the blood pressure until the effects of the depressant drug wear off. There is no specific antidote or reversal agent for the barbiturates. For the benzodiazepines (e.g., diazepam, midazolam [Versed]) a specific antagonist—Flumazenil (Mazicon)—is available. Reversal of narcotic effect is possible with naloxone hydrochloride (Narcan). It can be given intravenously—0.4 mg

(1 ml)—and is effective within 2 to 3 minutes. It may be repeated at 5- to 10-minute intervals if required. (When administered intramuscularly, the effect takes about 15 minutes.)

There is very rapid decay in the serum naloxone concentration; more than 90% of the original dose has left the serum within 5 minutes. There is also wide individual variation in disposition of naloxone.[43]

Drug Interactions Most depressant drugs used for IV sedation potentiate other depressants. It is essential to know what other drugs the patient is taking. Information concerning many drug interactions continues to be gathered at an ever-growing rate and ready reference should be available to the doctor.[44,45] In general, all CNS depressants interact to produce further depression—these include alcohol, barbiturates, sedatives, tranquilizers, antihistamines, narcotics, etc. Of particular concern for the dentist using these intravenous sedation techniques is the added caution for patients taking MAO inhibitors or the tricyclic antidepressants.

UNDERLYING MEDICAL ILLNESS

The initial patient history and evaluation will often indicate areas of concern prior to intravenous sedation. Patients with known hypersensitivity to the drugs to be used would not be subjected to this type of sedation. Alcoholics, narcotic addicts, and patients with underlying psychopathology should be assessed carefully before dental treatment.

In patients with advanced emphysema or chronic myocardial disease, one should avoid drugs that further depress pulmonary and cardiac function. Patients receiving adrenocorticosteroids may require an increase in perioperative steroid dosage to avoid adrenal crisis. In patients with acute narrow-angle glaucoma, diazepam and midazolam are contraindicated.

Older patients require very small doses of benzodiazepines for adequate sedation. Patients with chronic liver disease and the rare patient with intermittent porphyria tolerate barbiturates poorly. Hypothyroid patients deserve great caution with sedative and narcotic administration.

It is advisable for dentists who are not entirely familiar with the methods and potential complications of intravenous sedation to limit their patient selection to Class I and II risks—those without attendant serious medical illness.

A Newer Sedative Agent—Midazolam Hydrochloride

Midazolam hydrochloride (Versed), a water-soluble, short-acting imidazobenzodiazepine, is rapidly replacing diazepam as the principal intravenous sedative agent. In aqueous solution, it contains 5 mg/ml and is buffered to a pH of 3.3. At this acid pH, the benzodiazepine ring is open. After administration, at physiologic pH, the ring closes and produces its effects. Being acidic, it should not be mixed with alkaline solution.[46]

The primary advantage of midazolam is its lack of burning on administration and its very low incidence of phlebothrombosis. The drug undergoes hydroxylation by the liver and is excreted in the urine as a glucuronide conjugate. Midazolam fails to show a "second peak" effect, characteristic of diazepam, because midazolam's metabolites are inactive.[47] It is very rapidly distributed from the plasma, providing a brief duration of action. Its metabolism and excretion are significantly shorter than diazepam's with a metabolic half-life of approximately 2 hours, compared to greater than 24 hours for diazepam. Most of the midazolam binds to serum albumin.

In earlier studies of its effective dose range, 0.2 mg/kg was found to provide *general anesthesia* for 95% of the subjects.[48] Up to 0.6 mg/kg has been administered for general anesthesia without adverse effects. Anesthesia induction times varied from 1 to 2 minutes.

Conscious sedation is readily produced with slightly less than half of the sleep-inducing dose (0.07 to 0.09 mg/kg).[49] The total dose required for sedation for most adults is 2.5 to 7.5 mg, which shows wide individual variation and underscores the need for careful titration. Midazolam has two to three times the potency of diazepam. As with other benzodiazepines, elderly patients are more sensitive and require lower doses. Midazolam produces a dose-related anterograde amnesia that is even more pronounced than with diazepam or lorazepam.[50]

On the cardiovascular system midazolam causes slight reduction in blood pressure, but no dysrhythmias. At higher dosage, there is significant reduction in cerebral blood flow. Midazolam, like diazepam, causes equivalent respiratory depression. In studies of recovery a large dose (0.175 mg/kg) produced disorientation for 50 minutes, drowsiness for 81 minutes, and ataxia lasting 111 minutes.[51] (Intramuscularly, midazolam causes far less irritation and produces much greater amnesia than hydroxyzine).

Early clinical experience with midazolam used for sedation in dentistry has led to the recommendation that the ampule be diluted with sterile water immediately prior to injection to facilitate careful titration of a less concentrated solution.[52] A preferable aid in using midazolam is to draw up the 5 mg into a 1-ml tuberculin syringe. This serves to alert the operator to the potency of this agent.

Although midazolam was officially released for clinical practice in the United States in 1986, many clinical studies have confirmed significant advantages, primarily related to fewer venous complications, a shorter recovery period, and more profound amnesia.

Narcotics and Opioids

Narcotic medications have been a part of many conscious sedation techniques ever since their early introduction by Jorgensen. In essence, the experience with intravenous sedation drugs gained in hospital practice was applied (often uncritically) to the office situation. Without belaboring this issue much further, ambulatory or office sedation and anesthesia are "not better or worse than hospital practice, but they are surely different."[53]

Jorgensen's use of meperidine to augment his baseline barbiturate sedation was carefully calculated and specifically limited never to exceed 25 mg. White and Chang demonstrated that narcotic premedication prior to brief outpatient procedures reduced the recovery time by decreasing the dose of the hypnotic anesthetic re-

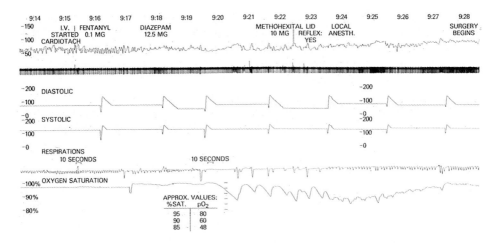

Fig. 7-11. Monitoring of chest excursions by pneumotachometer and oxygen saturation clearly shows the depressant effect of a narcotic added to the sedation regimen. Prolonged periods of apnea and hypoventilation lead to hypoxemia. (Courtesy Dr. SS Gelfman.)

quired.[54] Thus, narcotic premedication can be advantageous in the outpatient setting. There are other disadvantages that should be carefully weighed when considering the use of adjunctive narcotic medications.

Meperidine Hydrochloride (Demerol, Pethidine) Meperidine hydrochloride is available in 10 mg/ml, 25 mg/ml, and 50 mg/ml. Meperidine has sedative, analgesic and atropine-like effects, depending on dosage. Its onset of action, when administered intravenously, is 2 to 4 minutes and its duration of effect is 30 to 45 minutes.[8] The usual dose used as an adjunct in conscious sedation varies from 12.5 to 50.0 mg. There is no well-defined endpoint to evaluate its effect, short of respiratory depression. It is therefore usually given not by titration but by arbitrary estimate based on age, weight, etc. In lower doses it affords little analgesia but contributes to the sedative action of the primary drug(s) used in deepening the level of CNS depression. All narcotics depress respiration; all narcotics influence the baroreceptors in the aortic arch and carotid body, which may compromise compensatory reflexes and cause hypotension, especially in the ambulatory patient subject to rapid postural changes. All narcotics provoke nausea and vomiting, especially in the upright or ambulatory patient. Meperidine, in particular, provokes histamine release, which is usually a transient, local phenomenon but may lead to systemic release of histamine with sudden decrease in systemic vascular resistance and hypotension. Meperidine causes an increase in pulse rate and may precipitate some tachyarrhythmias. It is contraindicated in patients known to be allergic and is used with great caution in patients who are taking MAO inhibitors.

Pentazocine Hydrochloride (Talwin, Fortral) Introduced for parenteral use in 1967, pentazocine is a benzomorphan analgesic with some narcotic antagonist properties. At one point, this drug was widely used in conjunction with other sedative-hypnotic agents for conscious sedation. It has failed to live up to expectations, and its use has declined dramatically in recent years primarily because of its multiple adverse effects: a high incidence of neuropsychiatric effects including hallucinations, disorientation, bizarre feelings, vertigo, and frank psychosis.[55] Pentazocine causes more nausea and vomiting than morphine or meperidine. In therapeutic doses pentazocine produces as much respiratory depression as other narcotics.

Alphaprodine Hydrochloride (Nisentil) This drug is a rapid-acting narcotic analgesic with a short duration of action and with properties similar to meperidine and morphine. It has been used, particularly in children, for short procedures. Alphaprodine has been ''promoted'' for use by the pedodontist employing the submucosal route of administration. For adults, 0.4 to 0.6 mg is the usual dose. As with other narcotics, respiratory depression is an ever-present concern regardless of the route of administration. Restlessness, erroneously assumed to be an indication for drug, is more often an early manifestation of hypoxia, with the patient becoming disoriented and struggling to breathe more oxygen.

Fentanyl Citrate (Sublimaze) Originally introduced for IV sedation in combination with the long-acting sedative droperidol, this rapid-acting narcotic analgesic gradually replaced meperidine. Its major advantage was its reputed brief period of action. However, like all narcotics, fentanyl has significant respiratory depressant effects that may extend even beyond its 30 to 60 minutes of analgesic action. Respiratory depression has been noted to last for up to 4 hours in healthy volunteers.[56]

Another feature of this very potent narcotic—it is 100 times more potent than morphine (0.1 mg of fentanyl is equivalent to 10 mg of morphine and 100 mg of meperidine)—is its tendency to provoke chest wall rigidity, especially when administered rapidly. This complication requires controlled ventilation by the operator and may necessitate a muscle relaxant such as succinylcholine to overcome the resistance to ventilation of the lungs or reversal with naloxone. In an excellent paper Dionne et al. reported that cardiovascular and respiratory monitoring showed prolonged periods of apnea following the addition of fentanyl to diazepam sedation.[57] Stoeckel et al at the University of Bonn showed a biphasic effect of fentanyl on respiration with depression appearing later, secondary to a rise in plasma fentanyl concentration again almost 1 hour after its administration[58]; they cautioned against early discharge of the patient after receiving fentanyl. Goldberg et al cite chest wall rigidity with fentanyl, occurring in almost all patients prior to unconsciousness.[59] They have found sufentanil (Sufenta) to cause similar rigidity, which developed in the recovery room 3 hours later.

Hug and Murphy showed a similar prolonged effect of fentanyl in dogs, correlating cerebrospinal fluid concentration with respiratory depression that resulted in decreased ventilation and increased P_{CO_2}.[60] Early recovery was rapid but complete recovery was prolonged. Fentanyl was shown to be highly lipophilic. Repeated injections of fentanyl led to even greater accumulation and prolongation of depression.

Fentanyl was shown to have additive negative inotropic effects when used with diazepam.[61] Greenfield and Granada,[62] Kraut,[63] as well as others[64] have shown that the combination of diazepam, fentanyl, and minimal incremental methohexital regularly produces hypoxia—in the absence of adjunctive nasal oxygen. Although adding oxygen is beneficial, these patients still show elevated P_{CO_2}, indicative of continued respiratory depression.

Gelfman et al showed no significant enhancement of recovery when fentanyl was added to the sedation regimen consisting of diazepam and incremental methohexital.[65] The addition of a narcotic antagonist such as naloxone did result in a less prolonged recovery.[66] On a positive note, the use of fentanyl was judged by the operating surgeon to result in a more relaxed, cooperative patient who was less reactive to surgical stimuli.

Tomacheck et al studied the hemodynamic effects of varying doses of diazepam in conjunction with fentanyl.[66] Significant decreases of blood pressure were noted in those receiving the combination, compared to receiving fentanyl alone. This was attributed to a decrease in systemic vascular resistance.

More recently, newer, more potent congeners of fentanyl have been introduced: alfentanil citrate (Alfenta),[64, 67] sufentanil citrate, (Sufenta),[68] and the research drug carfentanil citrate are very rapidly acting and have different potencies than fentanyl. Alfentenil, a less potent analogue of fentanyl, appears to be a clinically superior adjuvant for outpatient anesthesia.[69] Alfentanil produces more intense respiratory depression than fentanyl and also causes less nausea and vomiting. Sufentanil is considerably more potent than fentanyl, whereas carfentanil is 800 times more potent than fentanyl!

Nevertheless, the adverse effects of these agents are typical of all opioids, including respiratory depression, skeletal muscle rigidity,[54] nausea and vomiting, occasional bradycardia, etc. These extremely potent agents should be reserved for use in patients who are intubated and have their respirations controlled.

Nalbuphine Hydrochloride (Nubain) This agent has properties that are best described as agonist/antagonist narcotic effects. In potency it is equivalent to morphine but lasts somewhat longer. It also produces side effects of drowsiness, sweaty and clammy feelings, nausea and vomiting, dizziness, and psychotomimetic effects including depression, dysphoria, confusion, and hallucinations reminiscent of pentazocine.[55] Its advantage may lie in the fact that the respiratory depression induced by nalbuphine plateaus at a given dose and does not intensify whereas morphine and other narcotics produce increasing depression with increasing dosage until apnea is produced.

Butorphanol Tartrate (Stadol) This drug is very similar to nalbuphine in that it produces both agonist and antagonist narcotic effects. It is five times more potent than morphine. It has a respiratory depression plateau effect similar to nalbuphine except that the depression caused by butorphanol is more prolonged. Untoward psychotomimetic effects are increased with higher dosages, and other adverse side effects occur.

Concerns Regarding Drug Combinations

The advent of intravenous medication for ambulatory office dentistry and oral surgery has been an important advance in the management of pain and anxiety. A primary concern of educators and knowledgeable practitioners is the safety associated with using potent drugs via the intravenous route. Various protocols and training criteria have been proposed to ensure the safe practice of intravenous sedation. Generally, emphasis is placed on the need to *titrate* these drugs slowly to avoid precipitous and unwarranted changes in cardiopulmonary and CNS status. Equally important is the operator's monitoring of vital signs and the awareness of even subtle changes that presage more adverse reactions.

The selection of a narcotic agent to be used along with diazepam, midazolam, or a short-acting barbiturate is well established in clinical practice. The origin of the choice of a narcotic seems to stem from two sources: (1) oral surgeons and others who have been trained in hospital operating rooms by physician anesthesiologists become very familiar and comfortable with the adjunctive use of narcotics in premedication and in the creation of neuroleptic, dissociative, and sedative states, and (2) another source of the selection of a narcotic is traceable to Niels Jorgensen, who pioneered conscious sedation in the office. His technique called for an initial titration with pentobarbital (Nembutal); then, depending on the amount of the barbiturate required to achieve a "baseline" of sedation, he added a small quantity of meperidine—not to exceed 25 mg. Dr. Jorgensen showed wisdom based on his extensive experience and respect for the potential adverse effects of the narcotic, especially in very susceptible individuals. Ultimately, he advised avoiding the narcotic in elderly patients and in those who showed significant medical compromise.

Transposing sedative and anesthetic techniques from the hospital operation room to the dental office, without modification, is fraught with potential hazards. Many differences exist in the methodologies of office anesthesia and sedation, which are based on valid criteria of patient selection, duration of operation, and depth of sedation required. One of these major differences between hospital and office anesthesia is the control of respiration. In the operating room, the airway is secured and respirations are controlled or assisted with the use of endotracheal intubation and a respirator. Rate and depth of respiration are closely monitored, and supplemental oxygen and other inhalational anesthetic agents are administered.

In most offices, intubation is rarely used. The integrity of the airway depends upon the physical maintenance of the jaw and tongue in a forward position, as held by the anesthesia assistant, and avoidance of foreign objects from blocking the airway as monitored by the surgeon and the surgical assistant. These techniques have been shown to be effective and safe when practiced by a competent office anesthesia team. Detractors who have not experienced outpatient anesthesia done successfully in this manner are reluctant to accept the results of several studies that show exceedingly low morbidity and mortality of office anesthesia, especially when compared to hospital anesthesia for comparable groups of patients undergoing elective operations.

However, for those practitioners not trained in general anesthesiology and unfamiliar with the management of the unconscious patients, deep sedation and general anesthesia are to be assiduously avoided.

In the absence of endotracheal intubation and controlled respirations, the patient is at greater potential risk of developing hypoxia. The growing availability of monitoring of oxygen saturation with pulse oximetry and carbon dioxide with capnography provides us with reliable and more rapid information concerning vital functions. In the past, in addition to monitoring the rate of respiration and some index of respiratory depth, we looked for the absence of cyanosis, tachycardia, and "restlessness," to avoid hypoxia. Electrocardiographic monitoring is now more widely used in office for deep sedation and general anesthesia. However, changes secondary to hypoxia may *not* become evident on the electrocardiogram until they have been present for several minutes.

Why *Not* to Use Narcotics for Ambulatory Sedation—a Polemic

Following are seven cogent reasons why *not* to use narcotics for ambulatory sedation, especially if the doctor is not prepared in general anesthesia practices.

1. *Narcotic analgesics have a profound effect on respiration.* This is so especially when they are combined with other CNS depressants. Numerous studies have shown that even in small quantities and when given intravenously, there is a significant decrease in Pao_2, an increase in $Paco_2$, and a decrease in pH, reflecting important changes in the physiology of respiration, cardiac, and brain functions. It has been pointed out that these changes are often not readily apparent in the clinical situation.

   After a medical legal review of a number of tragic "accidents" related to conscious sedation and ambulatory anesthesia, it is apparent that a common denominator of these complications was the use of intravenous narcotics coupled with a lack of appreciation of their profound effects.

   Greenfield and Granada,[62] Driscoll et al,[25] Dionne et al,[57] Gelfman et al,[65] Campbell et al,[64] Kraut,[63] and many others who have studied the respiratory depressant effects of even small quantities of narcotic added to sedative regimens confirm the changes in oxygen, carbon dioxide, and pH and recommend the adjunctive use of supplemental oxygen by nasal mask whenever narcotics are employed for intravenous sedation and anesthesia. Campbell et al recommend at least 35% to 40% oxygen whenever narcotic agents are used.[64]

Over the past 15 years, I have personally avoided the use of any opioid in my ambulatory conscious sedation cases. The use of narcotics, when indicated, was limited to general anesthesia cases when intubation and controlled respiration were employed in longer procedures. For short general anesthesia cases, intubation was not used; adjunctive oxygen was administered by nasal mask and special care for patency of the airway was maintained.

2. *Narcotics are primarily indicated to provide analgesia.* In all conscious sedation situations, the analgesic agent is the local anesthetic. We are fortunate in having excellent short-, moderate-, and long-duration local anesthetic agents that provide a very high incidence of freedom from pain secondary to surgery and other manipulations. An intravenous sedative is very helpful in enhancing the effect of the local anesthetic and relaxing the patient. There is no real need for a systemic analgesic agent if the local anesthetic is effective and if the potential hazard associated with the use of the intravenous narcotic is significant. The sedation that can be attained by using a narcotic can be readily and more safely attained by the use of an ataractic agent such as a benzodiazepine or a barbiturate. Thus, *using a narcotic represents the selection of the wrong drug for the wrong reason.*

3. *It is difficult to titrate the narcotic.* While *titration* of drugs is the keynote to safe and effective conscious sedation, it is extremely difficult to titrate narcotics because there are few reliable endpoints other than respiratory depression. Even large doses may not cause slurred speech or significant motor incoordination. At higher concentrations, pupillary constriction occurs as an excitatory action on the autonomic segment of the oculomotor nerve. Most practitioners give an "average dose" and therefore an arbitrary amount of narcotic, usually based on an estimate of the patient's weight, age, and

disposition. These criteria are based on the distribution curve, and the average dose does not consider the uniqueness of the individual being treated. The individual patient may well manifest extreme sensitivity to even a low dose of narcotic. I have known a number of such patients who give a history of "cardiac arrest" following a routine, average dose of meperidine and other narcotic agents. In one such patient, the need for postoperative analgesic medication prompted me to administer just 1 mg of morphine, intravenously, with some evident symptomatic relief of pain. A second 1-mg dose was followed by the development of hypotension, tachycardia, and a profound decrease in respiratory rate. The patient received no further narcotic analgesics. She was later found to have a familial history of sensitivity to narcotic agents.

4. *Narcotics produce an effect on the baroreceptors.* The effect is such that the blood pressure mechanism is less responsive to demands of positional changes. Narcotics produce arteriolar and venous dilation, which further serves to decrease blood pressure. This is particularly important in ambulatory patients who are expected to be able to leave the semisupine chair position and be discharged soon after completion of the procedure. In a hospital, the patient is transferred to a recovery room, while horizontal, and then goes back to bed for several hours. Most hospitals require that medicated patients be transported either on a gurney or at least seated in a wheelchair. Elderly patients are generally more susceptible to the development of postural hypotension, especially after receiving agents that depress baroreceptor function.

5. *Narcotics produce a fair incidence of nausea and vomiting.* Approximately 40% of ambulatory patients develop nausea and 20% develop vomiting after receiving narcotics.[70] Meperidine increases the sensitivity of the labyrinthine-vestibular

apparatus. These effects are often dose related, although some patients are much more susceptible than others, especially when they are moving about as ambulatory patients. Although the nausea and vomiting may be considered only a nuisance, they can be very distressing to the patient and may, in an obtunded patient, pose a real hazard of pulmonary aspiration.

6. *All narcotics produce histamine release.* Some narcotics produce more than others, but this may play a role in causing hypotension. Of greater concern is the precipitation of asthma and bronchospasm in susceptible patients. It is also recommended that meperidine be used with caution in patients with supraventricular tachycardias or atrial flutter. Its vagolytic action may produce a significant increase in ventricular response rate. Fentanyl, which is a very potent short-acting narcotic analgesic, shows depression of respiratory rate and depth that lasts *longer* than its analgesic effect. Histamine release is reportedly less common than with other narcotic analgesics, but it too can cause bronchoconstriction, chest wall rigidity, bradycardia, and most importantly, respiratory depression. The usual duration of effect is 30 to 60 minutes after a single dose of 0.1 mg fentanyl citrate intravenously, with a peak respiratory depressant effect that occurs 5 to 15 minutes after injection.

7. *Narcotics are invariably used as part of a multidrug regimen.* Data show that these techniques used in ambulatory conscious sedation are associated with a higher incidence of adverse reactions and complications. Effects are compounded and the depth of sedation is greater than is necessary to achieve a comfortable and cooperating patient who maintains consciousness and is free of anxiety and pain. Perhaps the singular significant advantage of the use of a narcotic for conscious intravenous sedation is the ability to specif-

ically reverse its effect with the narcotic antagonist naloxone.

In conclusion, the incorporation of a narcotic into ambulatory intravenous sedation is ill advised. Its disadvantages outweigh its contribution to sedation or analgesia. In the awake patient, the local anesthetic is a more effective analgesic agent. Titration of the narcotic based on individual tolerance is capricious. Narcotics all produce respiratory depression as well as depression of baroreceptor responsiveness to postural changes and have a significant incidence of nausea, vomiting, and release of histamine. Adjunctive oxygen via a nasal mask should be mandatory, as are clearance and competence of the oropharyngeal airway. Hypoventilation, induced by narcotics and aggravated by partial obstruction of the airway, invites disaster. Hypoxia remains the commonest cause of serious dysrhythmias and cerebral damage. "Restlessness" means "hypoxia," until it can be specifically ruled out by increasing the level of oxygen delivered to the brain.

Summary

Intravenous sedation offers the most accurate, effective, and safest way to sedate a patient. The endpoint should be a comfortable and cooperative patient whose pain is alleviated by the administration of regional local anesthesia. It requires a patient who understands the difference between being lightly sedated and not unconscious. Its primary purpose is to diminish anxiety and apprehension rather than to obtund protective reflexes. At all times, the patient remains conscious and appropriately responsive to question or command. This state can be readily achieved for most patients by carefully titrating a drug such as diazepam or midazolam. The use of multiple drugs is to be discouraged because it generally increases the level of sedation and the number of potential complications.

Titration should be individualized, rather than based on an arbitrary dose. The endpoint of titration is the patient's verbal acknowledgement that he or she feels more relaxed and shows subtle physical signs of such relaxation by postural and behavioral changes. The "Verrill sign" indicates a level of deep sedation, with attendant depression of the CNS that is too deep for most optimal cases of conscious sedation in the office setting.

Data are presented that strongly argue *against* the use of narcotics for office sedation. Appropriate preoperative, intraoperative, and postoperative monitoring is described to ensure safety and efficacy of the consciously sedated patient.[71]

References

1. Everett GB, Allen GD: Intravenous therapy—a review of site selection and technique, *Anesth Prog* 16(9):280-285, 1969.
2. Hecker JF, Lewis FBH, Stanley J: Nitroglycerin ointment as an aid to venipuncture, *Lancet* 1:332-333, 1983.
3. Jorgensen NB: Local anesthesia and intravenous premedication, *Anesth Prog* 13:168, 1966.
4. Hiatt W: The management of idiosyncrasy related to local anesthesia, *Anesth Prog* 16(5):133-137, 1969.
5. Richards RK, Smith NT, Katz J: The effects of interaction between lidocaine and pentobarbital on toxicity in mice and guinea pig atria, *Anesthesiology* 29:493-498, 1968.
6. Everett GB, Allen GD: Simultaneous evaluation of cardiorespiratory and analgesic effects of intravenous analgesia using pentobarbital, meperidine, and scopolamine with local anesthesia, *J Am Dent Assoc* 83:155-158, 1971.
7. Friend DB, McLemore GA: Medical progress: some abuses of drugs in therapy, *N Engl J Med* 254(6):1223-1230, 1956.
8. Rigg JRA, Ilsley AH, Verdig AE: Relationship of ventilatory response to steady-state blood pethidine concentrations, *Br J Anaesth* 53:613-620, 1981.
9. Flacke JW, Van Etten A, Flacke WE: Greatest histamine release from meperidine among 4 narcotics: double-blind study in man, *Anesthesiology* 59(3A):A51, 1983.
10. Newman MG et al: A comparative study of psychomotor effects of intravenous agents used in dentistry, *Oral Surg Oral Med Oral Pathol* 30(1):34-40, 1970.
11. Massumi RA et al: Ventricular fibrillation and tachycardia after intravenous atropine for treatment of bradycardias, *N Engl J Med* 287(7):336-338, 1972.
12. American Medical Association: *Drug evaluations,* Chicago, 1971, American Medical Association.
13. Shane SM: Intravenous amnesia for total dentistry in one sitting, *J Oral Surg* 24(1):27-32, 1966.
14. Foreman PA: Psychosedation: intravenous route. In McCarthy FM, editor: *Emergencies in dental practice, prevention and treatment,* ed 2, Philadelphia, 1972, WB Saunders.
15. Beer B et al: Cyclic adenosine monophosphate phosphodiesterase in brain: effect on anxiety, *Science* 176:428-430, 1972.
16. Wise CD, Berger BD, Stein L: Benzodiazepines: anxiety-reducing activity by reduction of serotonin turnover in the brain, *Science* 177:180-183, 1972.
17. Trieger N: Scientific abstract of The Medical Letter on Drugs and Therapeutics, 11(20):81-84, Oct 1969, *Anesth Prog* 17(1):15, 1970.
18. de Jong RH, Heavner JE: Diazepam prevents local anesthetic seizures, *Anesthesiology* 34:6, 1971.
19. Przbylan AC, Wang SC: *Pharmacologist* 9:2, 188, 1967. Quoted in *Valium (diazepam): pharmacology and brief clinical review,* Nutley, NJ, 1968, Hoffman-La Roche, Inc.
20. Geller E et al: The use of RO 15-1788: a benzodiazepine antagonist in the diagnosis and treatment of benzodiazepine overdose, *Anesthesiology* 61(3A):A135, 1984.
21. Grower MF, Russell EA, Jr, Getter L: Solubility of injectable valium in intravenous solutions, *Anesth Prog* 25(5):158-160, 1978.
22. Dalen JC et al: The hemodynamic and respiratory effects of diazepam (Valium), *Anesthesiology* 30 (3):259-263, 1969.
23. Gross JG, Smith L, Smith TC: Time course of ventilatory response to carbon dioxide after intravenous diazepam, *Anesthesiology* 57:18-21, 1982.
24. Jordan C et al: Respiratory depression following diazepam: reversal with high-dose naloxone, *Anesthesiology* 53:293-298, 1980.
25. Driscoll EJ et al: Sedation with intravenous diazepam, *J Oral Surg* 30(5):332-343, 1972.
26. O'Neill R et al: Intravenous diazepam in minor oral surgery, *Br Dent J* 128 (1):15-18, 1970.
27. Healy TES, Edmondson HD, Dudley Hall N: Intravenous diazepam in the mentally handicapped patient, *Br Dent J* 128(1):22-24, Jan. 1970.
28. Gregg JM, Ryan DE, Levin KH: The amnesic

actions of diazepam, *J Oral Surg* 32(9):651-664, 1974.

29. Gelfman SS et al: Conscious sedation with intravenous drugs: a study of amnesia, *J Oral Surg* 36(3):191-197, 1978.

30. Kaufman E et al: Analgesic action of intravenous diazepam, *Anesth Prog* 31(2):70-74, 1984.

31. Healy TEJ, Vickers MD: Laryngeal competence under diazepam sedation, *Proc Soc Med* 64(1):85-86, 1971.

32. Foreman PA, Neels R, Willetts PW: Diazepam in dentistry, *Anesth Prog* 15(9):253-258, Nov 1968.

33. Khosla VM, Boren W: Diazepam (Valium) as preoperative medication in oral surgery, *Oral Surg Oral Med Oral Pathol* 28:671-679, 1969.

34. Trieger N, Newman MG, Miller JG: An objective measure of recovery, *Anesth Prog* 16:4, 1969.

35. Newman MG, Trieger N, Miller JC: Measuring recovery from anesthesia—a simple test, *Anesth Analg* 48(1):136-140, 1969.

36. Newman MG, et al: A comparative study of psychomotor effects of intravenous agents used in dentistry, *Oral Surg Oral Med Oral Pathol* 30(1):34-40, 1970.

37. Baird ES, Hailey DM: Delayed recovery from a sedative: correlation of the plasma levels of diazepam with clinical effects after oral and intravenous administration, *Br J Anaesth* 44:803, 1972.

38. Letourneau JE, Denis R: The reliability and validity of the Trieger tests as a measure of recovery from general anesthesia in a day-care surgery unit, *Anesth Prog* 30(5):152-155, 1983.

39. Hoare AM: Pulmonary embolus after diazepam sedation, *J Am Med Assoc* 230(2):210, 1974.

40. Gelfman SS, Dionne RA, Driscoll EJ: Prospective study of venous complications following intravenous diazepam in dental outpatients, *Anesth Prog* 28(5):126-128, 1982.

41. Topazian RG: Accidental intra-arterial injections: a hazard of intravenous medication, *J Am Dent Assoc* 81(2):410-415, 1970.

42. Goldsmith D, Trieger N: Accidental intra-arterial injection: a medical emergency, *Anesth Prog* 22:180, 1975.

43. Actkenhead AR et al: Pharmacokinetics of intravenous naloxone in healthy volunteers, *Anesthesiology* 61(3A):A381, 1984.

44. Smith NT, Corbascio AN: *Drug interactions in anesthesia,* ed 2, Philadelphia, 1986, Lea & Febiger.

45. Smith NT, Miller RD, Corbascio AN: *Drug interactions in anesthesia,* Philadelphia, 1981, Lea & Febiger.

46. Dornauer RJ, Aston R: Update:midazolam maleate, a new water-soluble benzodiazepine, *J Am Dent Assoc* 106(5):650-652, 1983.

47. Peterson LJ: Clinical assessment of new IV sedation agents and techniques, *J Dent Res* 63(6):838-841, 1984.

48. Reves JG, Kissin L, Smith LR: The effective dose of midazolam, *Anesthesiology* 55:82, 1981.

49. Aun C et al: A comparison of midazolam and diazepam for intravenous sedation in dentistry, *Anesthesiology* 39:589-593, 1984.

50. Dundee JW: Updating the benzodiazepines, *SAAD Digest* 5(7):169-171, 1984.

51. Fragen RJ, Caldwell NJ: Recovery from midazolam used for short operations, *Anesthesiology* 53(3):S11, 1980.

52. Parsons JD: Some observations on the use of midazolam in conscious sedation, *SAAD Digest* 5(9):220-222, 1984.

53. Trieger N: Not better nor worse, just different, *Anesth Prog* 27(2):44, 1980 (editorial).

54. White PF, Chang T: Effect of narcotic premedication on the intravenous anesthetic requirement, *Anesthesiology* 61 (3A):A389, 1984.

55. Abramowitz M: Reevaluation of parenteral pentazocine, *Med Lett* 18(11):46-47, 1976.

56. Malamed SF: *Sedation: a guide to patient management,* St Louis, 1989, Mosby-YearBook.

57. Dionne RW et al: Cardiovascular and respiratory response to intravenous diazepam, fentanyl, methohexital in dental outpatients, *J Oral Surg* 39(5):343-349, 1981.

58. Stoeckel H et al: Plasma fentanyl concentrations and occurrence of respiratory depression in volunteers, *Br J Anaesth* 54:1087-1095, 1982.

59. Goldberg M et al: Postoperative rigidity following sufentanil administration, *Anesthesiology* 63(2):199-201, 1985.

60. Hug CC, Murphy MR: Fentanyl disposition in cerebrospinal fluid and its relationship to ventilatory depression in the dog, *Anesthesiology* 50:342-349, 1979.

61. Reeves JG, Kissin J, Fournier SE: Additive negative inotropic effect of a combination of diazepam and fentanyl, *Anesthesiology* 59(3):A326, 1983.

62. Greenfield W, Granada MG: The use of narcotic antagonist in the anesthetic management of the ambulatory oral surgery patient, *J Oral Surg* 32:760-766, 1974.

63. Kraut RA: Continuous transcutaneous O_2 and CO_2 monitoring during conscious sedation for oral surgery, *J Oral Maxillofac Surg* 43:489-492, 1985.

64. Campbell RL et al: Respiratory effects of fentanyl, diazepam and methohexital sedation, *J Oral Surg* 37:555-562, 1979.

65. Gelfman SS et al: Recovery following intravenous sedation during dental surgery performed under local anesthesia, *Anesth Analg* 59(10): 775-781, 1980.

66. Tomacheck RC et al: Diazepam-fentanyl interaction: hemodynamic and hormonal effects in coronary surgery, *Anesth Anal* 62:881-884, 1983.

67. Rosow CE et al: Alfentanil and fentanyl in short surgical procedures, *Anesthesiology* 59(3): A345, 1983.

68. Abramowitz M: Sufentanyl—a new opioid anesthetic, *Med Lett* 26:675, 106, 1984.

69. Coe V, Shafer A, White PF: Techniques for administering alfentanil during outpatient anesthesia—a comparison with fentanyl, *Anesthesiology* 59(3):A347, 1983.

70. Shaefer A et al: Outpatient premedication: use of midazolam and opioid analgesics, *Anesthesiology* 71:495-501, 1989.

71. Trieger N: Intravenous sedation in dentistry and oral surgery, *Int Anesthesiol Clin* 27:2. 83-91, 1989.

8

General Anesthesia: Ambulatory and In-Hospital

Outpatient general anesthesia for dental treatment has achieved an enviable record of safe performance over the past 35 years in the United States and other countries. Prior to the introduction of intravenous barbiturates the principal means of rendering a patient unconscious for brief periods was nitrous oxide gas. There are records available that attest to the great skill and dexterity possessed by older confreres who were able to use this anesthetic to perform even lengthy procedures in the dental office. However, the beginnings of ambulatory dental anesthesia with the use of the intravenous barbiturate hexobarbital (Evipal) were first reported in the American literature in an article by Edward C. Thompson in 1935.[1] His professional association with Berto A. Olson of Hollywood favored the future development of intravenous anesthesia in Southern California. A short while later John Lundy brought thiopental sodium (Pentothal) to the Mayo Clinic, and it proved to be a better drug than hexobarbital. Adrian Hubbell took this drug and technique from the Mayo Clinic back to Southern California, where he further refined methods of its administration. Drs. Hubbell, Krogh, and others, such as S. L. Drummond-Jackson in the United Kingdom, taught its application for office practice for many years to members of the dental profession. Hubbell cited his successful experiences with over 250,000 intravenous anesthesias to office patients.[2]

It is to these early pioneers and to some of their stalwart contemporaries that we and our patients owe a debt of gratitude. Only recently has it become appropriate for many medical anesthesiologists[3,4] to endorse the ambulatory use of general anesthetics, faced as they are with the tighter control of hospital beds and the rising costs of hospitalization. They are learning to "dog-ear" a page from the textbook of the oral surgeon who forgoes the use of heavy premedication, deep general anesthesia, tracheal intubation, and prolonged recovery.

The patient who walks into the oral surgeon's office must walk out again after undergoing anesthesia and surgery of relatively short duration. The depth of anesthesia required for such operations is shallow, with the surgeon and his or her team geared to work efficiently on a patient who may be responding to the surgical stimulation by moving and even phonating. Amnesia is marked and patients are uniformly pleased with the experience. The requirements for ambulatory anesthesia in dentistry often differ considerably from those for inpatient anesthesia: profound muscular relaxation is not required. The use of local analgesia enables the operator to work at extremely light levels, which are aimed at producing a decrease in anxiety and apprehension, and amnesia for the event. A primary hazard for the ambulatory patient undergoing light anesthesia without tracheal intubation is the vulnerability of the airway. Dentists work in the airway and must exercise continuous caution to ensure its patency in the obtunded or unconscious patient.

A growing tendency in office dental anesthesia is the use of agents that produce the desired effects without unconsciousness: there are

123

many patients who can easily tolerate procedures under sedative and tranquilizing drugs while remaining conscious, who a few years ago would have been subjected to complete anesthesia.

Although there are many nuances to the practice of ambulatory anesthesia, most offices rely upon intravenous barbiturates for adults and inhalation anesthesia with nitrous oxide and halothane for children.

Inhalation Anesthesia

HALOTHANE (FLUOTHANE)

Halothane (2-bromo-2-chloro-1:1:1-trifluorothane) is a potent inhalational anesthetic that has been extensively used over the past 30 years for outpatient anesthesia in dentistry. Its potency and safety are well documented.[5-10] Whether used alone or in combination with a barbiturate administered intravenously, halothane provides an excellent adjunct to oral surgical and general dental anesthetic management. With halothane-oxygen at 2% to 3% concentration, induction varies from 2 1/2 to 6 minutes; excitement or agitation rarely occurs and restraints are not necessary.[10] In the unpremedicated patient, halothane-oxygen anesthesia provides reliable signs and symptoms of anesthetic progress and depth. Eye signs, respirations, heart rate, blood pressure, and relaxation of the jaw all readily identify the appropriate level for surgical intervention.

The heart rate is particularly helpful in gauging anesthetic depth; should bradycardia occur, it is readily reversible by reducing the inspired concentration of halothane. A decrease in blood pressure invariably develops in patients under halothane when a surgical plane of anesthesia is reached. Physiologically, a lowering of blood pressure in these circumstances may be regarded as a safety feature; the heart can do "volume work" better than "pressure work." With the decrease in cardiac output that accompanies all anesthetics, the myocardium of the patient receiving halothane is not being called upon to work against a high-pressure gradient, and hence, the patient remains well oxygen-

ated, warm, and distinctly free of shocklike symptoms despite the lowered systolic and diastolic pressures.

Patients should be inducted to a surgical plane of anesthesia before operative intervention. When the eyes have become fixed and centered and the pupils constricted, the jaw will be relaxed; placing a bite block is then easily done without forceful opening of the mouth. Although surgery can be started before this level of relaxation is reached, it is not recommended except for the briefest operations. The patient is still in the excitement stage of anesthesia and will react to painful stimuli with gross movements and phonation.

When an intravenous barbiturate, for example methohexital sodium (Brevital), is used for anesthetic induction, followed by inhalation with halothane for anesthetic maintenance, the chief advantage is a greatly shortened induction time, which most adult patients prefer. It is also especially desirable for patients who will not tolerate a mask while awake.

Rarely is halothane-oxygen used alone. Clinically, nitrous oxide is added to the mix to obtain an enhanced concentration effect because of its low blood solubility. It results in an increase in effective alveolar ventilation and also produces the "second gas" effect.[11] With the increase in ventilation, there is an increased uptake of halothane or other volatile agents. The price paid for the use of nitrous oxide to enhance induction is seen in the higher incidence of excitement in the unpremedicated patients. This is also confirmed by animal studies.[12] Although this excitement period is fairly short, the patient may need to be restrained during this interval, whereas with halothane-oxygen alone the excitement period is both brief and readily controlled without restraints.

Recovery from halothane is relaxed and fairly short. With most brief surgical procedures the recovery time will be only slightly longer than the induction time.

Adjunctive local anesthetics containing 1:100,000 epinephrine are used with caution. The total amount is limited to less than 0.2 mg (equivalent to approximately 10 dental cartridges containing a 1:100,000 concentration of epinephrine), and each injection is done with careful aspiration to avoid intravascular placement. It has been shown that relatively large amounts of epinephrine are required to induce arrhythmias in patients under halothane anesthesia.[13,14] Karl et al concluded that children tolerate higher doses of epinephrine than adults during halothane anesthesia, and they advise that at least 10 μg/kg of epinephrine may be safely used.[15]

As a potent anesthetic, halothane has largely replaced other, less effective inhalational agents, such as Vinethene and Trilene, particularly in children. Recent literature reviews of some of the "apparent" cases of liver necrosis associated with halothane have found a number of them to be without justification or confirmation.[16,17] Unfortunately, earlier reports have discouraged many practitioners from using this general anesthetic.

Rarely would the dentist-anesthesiologist become aware of any delayed complications arising from the administration of halothane; not only are they very infrequent but also these untoward effects generally do not manifest themselves until at least 1 week postoperatively and sometimes several weeks later. Only the most perceptive patient would associate his or her symptoms with a dental visit several weeks before. It is conceivable that a patient would go to a physician and, despite a thorough history, not reveal a recent anesthetic administration.

Halothane and Hepatic Dysfunction Current concern with the development of hepatitis associated with the use of halothane deserves further comment.* Since the introduction of halothane in the United Kingdom in 1956 and 2 years later in the United States, it attained wide popularity as an "ideal" anesthetic agent. In 1963, though, reports relating it to hepatic dysfunction began to appear. This was not unexpected, considering our previous experiences

with chloroform and other halogenated agents. Noteworthy is the fact that although halothane was used for about 80% to 90% of anesthesias in the United Kingdom,[18] dissatisfaction was reported predominantly in the United States where only 50% to 60% of all anesthetic administration employed halothane.

A major reason for this can be found in the literature of Little.[19] He states that the first nine papers reporting liver damage following halothane administration, including the three in 1963 that attracted most interest, appeared in the United States. Because these cases subsequently drew attention in the lay press, many individuals not fully trained in anesthesia, including physicians, became aware of the problem. With many people having an appreciation of only the superficial details, the dilemma grew out of proportion.

Even with the reassuring conclusions of the National Halothane Study,[16] complacency about the issue became difficult as more and more reports appeared. This was highlighted by Klatskin and Kimberg, who provided proof that halothane hepatitis does actually exist.[20] Their case involved an anesthesia resident who was exposed almost daily to halothane. During his training he suffered recurrent episodes of hepatitis. Each relapse coincided with his return to work and re-exposure to the anesthetic. Deliberate rechallenge with halothane led to chills and fever. A liver biopsy showed the histologic features of hepatitis and hepatocellular necrosis, which eventually led to scarring and cirrhosis. Because a liver biopsy was not performed at the onset of the illness, the possibility of a preexisting cirrhosis cannot be ruled out. However, the results following re-exposure to halothane strongly implicate it as the etiologic agent.

National Halothane Study Controversy within the profession stimulated the formation of a committee in 1963 by the National Academy of Sciences' National Research Council to study the problem. The resultant National Halothane Study was released in 1966, with a final report in 1969.[16]

The study was retrospective in style, covering anesthetic administration in 34 institutions dur-

---

*Portions of this section are reprinted from Trieger N and Rubinstein S: The current status of halothane, *J Oral Surg* 31:595-599, 1973.

ing the years 1959 to 1962. A total of about 850,000 cases were studied; of these, 250,000 patients received halothane. A total of 82 cases of fatal hepatic necrosis were discovered, which occurred within 6 weeks of surgery. All but 9 could be explained from causes other than anesthesia. These were attributed to the following:

1. The patient's known disease
2. Postoperative complications
3. Shock
4. Hypoxia
5. The surgical procedures

Seven of the nine patients received halothane. Thus, at worst the incidence of fatal hepatic necrosis in this study was 7 out of 250,000, or about 1 in 35,000.

The committee's conclusions were as follows:

1. Fatal hepatic necrosis following anesthesia was a rare occurrence.
2. The contribution of halothane to such fatalities, while not ruled out, was an even rarer phenomenon.
3. Halothane was a safe anesthetic because the overall mortality following its use was 1.87%, compared to an average of 1.93% for all anesthetic procedures.

This information indicated that halothane appeared to be no worse and, in many instances, a better anesthetic agent than others by comparison. In a recent study by Fisher et al halothane was compared with enflurance and isoflurane and was found to be the agent of choice for children undergoing short "ambulatory" procedures.[17]

Diagnosis of Halothane Hepatitis   Klion, Schaffner, and Popper have attempted to define the clinical course of halothane hepatitis as observed in 32 patients.[21] The first abnormal event is usually fever developing not less than 7 days after the first exposure, with a range of 8 to 14 days, and usually accompanied by malaise and gastrointestinal symptoms such as right-sided upper abdominal pain. After several exposures, fever is noted 1 to 11 days postoperatively. Jaundice appears soon after the pyrexia, about 10 to 28 days after the first insult, but with multiple exposures about 3 to 17 days later. In their stud-

ies, the authors found the white blood count usually normal, but sometimes an eosinophilia was present.

Although at first glance this description appears diagnostic, the majority of authorities[21-25] believe that hepatic dysfunction associated with halothane has no particular manifestations that differentiate it from other causes of liver damage. As Trey et al point out, postoperative fever is as common after the use of other anesthetics as it is after halothane.[26] Likewise, postoperative jaundice is of little prognostic value concerning the outcome of subsequent exposures because it can occur from a variety of other sources, including blood transfusions, various drugs used in modern clinical medicine, operative procedures, septicemia, shock, and coincident viral hepatitis. More than 50,000 cases of infectious hepatitis are reported annually, and an even greater number of cases of serum hepatitis occur after the administration of blood and blood products.[24] Simpson, Strumin, and Walton, quoting Dykes and Bunker, indicate that some 200 to 300 patients each year are likely to be subjected to anesthesia while incubating viral hepatitis.[27]

Mechanism of Action of Halothane Hepatitis

With no unique clinical signs or morphologic patterns to identify halothane hepatitis, the next step for investigators was to try to define a biochemical basis for its production. Some possible mechanisms have been postulated. It is generally accepted that neither halothane nor its final metabolites—bromide, chloride, and trifluoroacetic acid—are hepatotoxic. Bromide and chloride in the amounts produced by clinical concentrations of halothane administration are not harmful because these elements can enter the normal pathways of metabolism. Similarly, trifluoroacetic acid, which is eliminated by way of the urine, would have to accumulate in great quantities, which are not reached in clinical practice, in order to cause liver damage.

In the metabolism of halothane to trifluoroacetic acid, intermediate metabolites are formed. One theory suggests that because of the free valent form, the compound that forms is highly reactive, and it is possible for it to combine with mitochondria in the liver. The resultant combination could impair normal reactions and specifically interfere with normal cellular metabolism and release of needed constituents. With prolonged action of these nonfunctional complexes, hepatocellular damage could occur.

Another possibility concerning the intermediary metabolite is that once it combines with mitochondria, this grouping may then act as an antigen, similar to chlorpromazine combining with mitochondria to act as a hapten. Because the major metabolic pathway of halothane is in the liver, it is reasonable to assume that hepatocellular damage may result as part of an immunologic response. Antimitochondrial antibodies have been identified in cases of halothane hepatitis, but they are not specific because they are also found in patients with primary biliary cirrhosis, chronic active hepatitis, viral hepatitis, certain connective tissue disorders, and after administration of certain drugs, such as chlorpromazine.[22,28] An increase in the results of the lymphocyte stimulation test in patients with halothane hepatitis has been shown by Paronetto and Popper[29]; however, it was subsequently shown that surgery and anesthesia normally depress the lymphocyte production, which then rebounds several days postoperatively.[28]

If we assume the validity of an intermediary metabolite as the causative agent in halothane hepatitis, it then becomes necessary to discuss the possibilities that may either potentiate its action or result in its elimination; any one of a number of factors that have an influence on this intermediary substance could be capable of determining hepatic injury. One such possibility revolves about the enzyme system concerned with the breakdown of halothane. These enzymes are concentrated in the endoplasmic reticulum, with their highest concentration in the liver. Many drugs, including anesthetic agents, have the capacity of increasing the amount of endoplasmic reticulum and, in turn, the quantity of enzymes. Because these enzymes last for several weeks, individuals receiving closely spaced halothane administrations would have the capacity to cope with increases in the intermediary metabolite.

This leads to a discussion concerning multiple exposures at short intervals. It is a widely accepted practice to use another anesthetic if the patient has received halothane in the recent past. Practitioners who follow this concept base this practice on the fact that closely spaced exposures might result in the production of greater amounts of intermediary metabolites than can be coped with by the body. With reference to the previous theory, it should be kept in mind that it is difficult to evaluate an individual's ability of enzyme induction; this accounts for the fact that rare patients develop hepatitis when exposed repeatedly to halothane, whereas others sustain no ill effects. With this in mind, it is recommended policy to refrain from using halothane again within a 3-month period. This is said to ensure complete elimination of the agent from the body.[17,22,23] Bruce insists, however, that there are no data to support the contention that halothane should be given no more often than every 3 months.[25]

Vergani et al showed that serum samples from patients with halothane-associated fulminant hepatic failure reacted specifically with halothane-altered liver cells from rabbits.[30] Specific antibodies to cell membranes were demonstrated by immunofluorescence and cytotoxicity techniques, suggesting an immunologic component to this condition. Dienstag finds that "rare hepatotoxicity not withstanding, halothane is a safe anesthetic whose advantages far outweigh its potential dangers. Susceptibility is increased in adults, obese persons, and females.[31] He offers an alternative interpretation of Vergani's data and proposes that the etiology is one of "idiosyncrasy" rather than "hypersensitivity."

More recently it has been demonstrated in rats that hypoxia plays a significant role in the occurrence of hepatitis associated with anesthetic agents, especially halothane.[32,33]

Another factor that tends to prolong the presence of halothane is body weight. Halothane has an affinity for lipids and tends to accumulate in fat deposits throughout its administration. Thus, whereas a normal patient might be able to cope with the anesthetic, the liver of an obese individual or a chronically ill, debilitated, or starved patient with a "fatty" liver would be subjected to a larger quantity of the drug over a longer period of time.

The duration of anesthesia is the last factor to be considered in regard to potentiation of the effect of halothane. It may require a long period of time for a fixed amount of halothane to be metabolized in accordance with the concept of enzyme saturation, resulting in a prolonged period for its complete elimination from the body.

Discussion Simpson, Strumin, and Walton estimate that 50 million halothane anesthetics had been administered up to 1971.[27] The occurrence of hepatitis resulting from the use of halothane must be acknowledged, but its prominence and prevalence have been exaggerated.

Today halothane is used in dental offices for ambulatory anesthesia because of its many good qualities, including potency, ease of control, and rapidity of induction and recovery, all of which far outweigh its infrequent hazards. Since many patients treated in this manner are of pediatric age, its continued use is recommended. Solosko, Frissell, and Smith reported on the lack of adverse effects in a child who received 111 halothane anesthesias over a 10-year period.[34] More recently, however, Lewis and Blair reported a case of halothane-associated hepatitis in a 3-year-old who received four halothane anesthesias over a 5-month period and showed positive antibodies to rabbit hepatocytes previously sensitive to halothane.[35]

Carney and Van Dyke in their critical review point out that after 13 years of use only 11 cases of possible pediatric halothane hepatitis were seen.[22] This probably relates to the ability of young livers to produce the metabolic enzymes and cope with the ensuing insult more easily. Children (0 to 9 years of age) represent 12% of the surgical population and receive halothane for 91% of their operations.

Up to the present time we have not experienced any case reports relating hepatitis resulting from in-office administration of halothane. This could be due to the fact that patients undergoing elective dental procedures are not subjected to the same contributing factors that cause liver damage, which are found in patients undergoing more extensive general surgery. Most dental operations under halothane anesthesia are of relatively short duration, with the preponderance of patients being young. Halothane in these circumstances is a choice anesthetic. This view may be at variance with the opinion of many who believe that halothane should be reserved for major surgery.

Patients receiving halothane must be followed carefully during the postoperative period, with particular concern for the development of otherwise unexplained fever or jaundice. They should be specifically advised to report any such symptoms.

An analogy between halothane and penicillin suggests itself at this point. Despite the fact that 6% to 10% of the population report allergy to penicillin and an estimated 300 to 1000 related deaths from penicillin anaphylaxis occur each year in the United States,[36] no one has seriously suggested doing away with penicillin even though other antibiotics are available. It is just too valuable and effective when used properly in patients who are screened by a careful medical history.

Halothane is an excellent agent for office use, and it would be unfortunate if it were discontinued in favor of older agents such as divinyl ether and trichloroethylene, both of which have serious shortcomings. Halothane has already achieved the distinction of being a tried and true agent and should not be dismissed from regular use for ambulatory anesthesia. It continues to compare very favorably against newer inhalation agents.[17]

ENFLURANE (ETHRANE)

Enflurane is a 2-chloro-1,1,2-trifluoroethyl difluoromethyl ether. This agent is a potent inhalational anesthetic related to halothane and methoxyflurane. It was extensively studied prior to its release for clinical use in late 1972 by the Food and Drug Administration. Because of its potency it provides a rapid induction and recovery. Concentrations for induction are higher than with halothane; generally 4% to 6% enflurane is required to induct an unpremedicated patient within a reasonable period of time, that is, 4 to 5 minutes. Maintenance levels may run 2% to 3% in the nonintubated patient. Although cardiac rates and rhythms remain stable, blood pressures tend to decrease with increasing depth of anesthesia. Deep levels of enflurane anesthesia are characterized by EEG changes of high voltage, fast frequency, and spike-dome complexes reminiscent of seizure activity. These may be associated with twitching or jerking. No associated hepatic or renal problems have been reported with the use of enflurane so far.[37-40]

In a study on outpatients by Trieger and Lasner, enflurane was found to be an effective, readily controllable, and safe anesthetic for outpatient use.[40] When enflurane was compared with intravenous anesthetics (diazepam and methohexital), recovery times as determined by the modified Bender Motor Gestalt (Trieger Dot Test) did not differ significantly. The anticipated slowing of the heart rate that is seen with halothane was not experienced with enflurane. Increasing anesthetic depth is readily assessed by clinical observation of muscular relaxation, classical Guedel eye signs, nonreactivity to painful stimuli, and blood pressure changes.

METHOXYFLURANE (PENTHRANE)

A light level of anesthesia with this anesthetic agent produces analgesia. Methoxyflurane is a very potent inhalation anesthetic. Because of its extremely high blood and brain solubility, induction and recovery are prolonged. Another concern is the remarkable uptake of methoxyflurane by the rubber hoses, tubes, and masks, requiring greater concentrations to achieve induction. One worker observed that he had to first "put his anesthesia machine to sleep" before he could anesthetize his patient. It is recommended that plastic tubings and masks replace rubber goods when methoxyflurane is used. Recovery from methoxyflurane anesthesia is very slow, and therefore it has a limited place in outpatient anesthesia.

Renal toxicity has been reported following the use of methoxyflurane; symptomatically, there is a high-volume, low-specific-gravity urine flow with hypernatremia and elevated blood urea nitrogen. These effects are dose related and do not appear when smaller doses and shorter exposures are experienced.[41]

Goldstein, Dragon, and Cobb used methoxyflurane for its analgesic property in 35 conscious patients.[42] Some analgesia was achieved in almost all patients but was judged to be satisfactory in only 20%.

TRICHLOROETHYLENE

This agent had been widely used for short procedures in outpatient anesthesia. It has a number of significant drawbacks that should discourage its continued use. In the presence of soda lime trichloroethylene decomposes to hydrochloric acid and phosgene, which are both toxic agents. It is usually administered in a nonrebreathing system via a vaporizer with a wick capable of delivering high vapor concentrations. Toxicity has been related to degradation products such as dichloroacetylene, which produces transient sensory defects particularly involving the trigeminal nerves.

Because of its high blood and brain solubility (similar to methoxyflurane), induction would tend to be prolonged. Again, like methoxyflurane, recovery is longer than with halothane. The breakdown products of trichloroethylene include trichloroacetic acid and trichloroethanol (the active ingredient of the hypnotic drug chloral hydrate). Breakdown products are detected up to 1 week after administration. Under trichloroethylene anesthesia, jaw relaxation is poor and laryngeal reflexes may remain active, although its analgesic effect is good. Attempts to deepen anesthesia present one of the major hazards to its use; cardiac irregularities may be precipitated, especially if there is attendant hypoxia or hypercapnia or if adrenalin has been injected.[43] Trichloroethylene offers an advantage in being very inexpensive and was used for brief procedures in younger children as an adjunct to nitrous oxide–oxygen anesthesia. However, better, more reliable, and safer agents are preferable.

ISOFLURANE (FORANE)

Isoflurane (1-chloro-2,2,2,trifluoroethyl difluoromethyl ether) is a clear, colorless, pungent, noninflammable, potent inhalation anesthetic. Induction by mask in an unpremedicated patient is often associated with excitement, coughing, breath-holding, or laryngospasms. Under isoflurane anesthesia, the skin remains pink, warm, and dry with the pupils constricted and centrally fixed. Pharyngeal and laryngeal reflexes are obtunded and respirations are depressed. Tidal volume decreases, although ventilatory rate actually increases. Despite this increase in rate, ventilatory assistance is necessary to compensate for the depression.

Cardiac rate tends to be maintained or moderately increased despite the depth of anesthesia, while blood pressure decreases with increasing depth. Heart rhythm is quite stable during isoflurane anesthesia, with a greater resistance to epinephrine-induced dysrhythmias than with halothane. Isoflurane anesthesia, unlike enflurane, causes no evidence of irritation to the central nervous system (CNS). Its biotransformation is less than with either halothane or enflurane, and it has not been associated with hepatic toxicity to date.[44,45]

For induction, 3% to 3.5% vaporized in oxygen or in nitrous oxide–oxygen mixture is used. Maintenance dosage varies from 0.5% to 3% (slightly higher when nitrous oxide is not used). An accurately calibrated vaporizer must be used.

PREOXYGENATION (DENITROGENATION)

It is standard practice when initiating general anesthesia to have the patient breathe oxygen initially for approximately 4 to 5 minutes to achieve nitrogen washout.[45] Within 2 minutes of breathing 100% oxygen, over 95% of the nitrogen is displaced and the partial pressure of oxygen in the blood rises significantly. This is thought to create a buffer or safety margin against any subsequent hypoxia during induction, intubation, etc.

In a recent study, four deep breaths of 100% oxygen were shown to achieve the same PaO_2 (350 mm Hg) as 5 minutes of spontaneous breathing of 100% oxygen.[46] Thus there appears to be no need to "denitrogenate" the patient for 3 to 5 minutes.

Patient Positioning in Ambulatory Anesthesia

There has been considerable discussion about the position of the patient relative to both airway maintenance and cardiovascular function. Bourne insisted that one of the greatest hazards for the patient seated upright in a dental chair is unrecognized fainting (syncope).[47] He attributed most of the anesthetic catastrophes in dental offices to the patient fainting while receiving a general anesthetic. His strong recommendation was to maintain the dental patient in a supine position. Allen[48] and others[49] point out that the semisupine position is much better than the fully supine in regard to airway control and cardiovascular functions. In the fully supine position cardiac output, total peripheral resistance, and blood pressure decline, whereas in the semisupine posture the cardiac output increases in response to the decline in total peripheral resistance.[49] It also allows the lungs to achieve greater compliance when the abdominal viscera are not pushing backward against the diaphragm and limiting excursion. Most oral surgeons prefer to work with the patient's head up at an angle of 30 to 40 degrees and with the legs straight out or slightly elevated.

A study of physiologic changes secondary to patient positioning confirmed that the upright sitting posture is least desirable and that the semireclining position at a 45-degree angle is best for office anesthesia procedures. In the upright position, with the legs down, subjects receiving methohexital showed an increased blood pressure, an increased and then a decreased heart rate, and a slowing of venous return from the extremities. Breathing efficiency was, however, excellent in the sitting position. Extending the legs did not significantly improve the cardiovascular changes.

By contrast, in the semireclining position, venous return was favorable and cardiac output was well maintained. Breathing efficiency was favorable.

In the head-down position, blood pressure decreased and heart rate increased while decreased breathing was compensated for by an increased blood supply to the lungs. Additional intravenous anesthesia led to depressed respiration and evidence of myocardial depression, with a decrease in cardiac output attributed to the direct effect of the drug on the heart. Also noted in this study was that three of the volunteers fainted while sitting in the upright position. Of special note was that their physiologic parameters remained abnormal for more than 1 hour after fainting.[50]

The significance of fainting is well demonstrated by Allen, who showed that it requires almost 2 hours for parameters of cardiovascular function to return to normal after fainting.[43] He advised that further anesthesia or surgery should be delayed or even deferred to another day. Generally, dental and oral surgical procedures are elective in the sense that they are not essential to sustain life. Discretion dictates that adverse reactions be considered as an important indication to curtail or postpone the anticipated surgery.

Intravenous Anesthesia For the Ambulatory Patient

Intravenous thiopental (Pentothal) 2.5% and methohexital (Brevital) 1% are the mainstays of ambulatory anesthesia practice. For most oral surgical procedures performed in the office, they provide a rapid, pleasant induction, ease of administration, and satisfactory anesthesia for relatively short periods. They avoid "the progressive dementia experienced with inhalational agents."[47]

Most office dental surgical procedures, such as removal of teeth or incision and drainage of an abscess, may require an operating time that varies from less than 1 minute to 20 to 30 minutes. When these intravenous techniques are used by a well-trained office team, their efficacy and safety are easily established. In Driscoll's 1966 study, the morbidity and mortality reported by 1000 U.S. oral surgeons using general anesthesia were found to be 1 death in 315,000 cases.[51] Allen cites a study conducted in Los Angeles County with a zero mortality in over 6,000,000 Brevital administrations and compares this experience with 1 death in 11,266 hospital anesthesias given for tonsillectomy operations.[48] However, these highly satisfactory

records are marred by being incomplete; they do not reflect the total experience of all patients so treated. Nevertheless, the record is an enviable one for dental outpatient anesthesia. Further statistics gathered by the American Association of Oral and Maxillofacial Surgeons showed that 117 members of the Southern California group had a mortality rate associated with office anesthesia of 1 in 432,000 anesthesias.[52,53] In Massachusetts (1980) over a 3-year period, 157 members reported an incidence of 1 in 1,176,660 anesthesias. In 1981, in the state of Ohio, experience by dentists and oral surgeons having special anesthesia permits, over a 7-year period, was 1 in 750,000; two fatalities occurred in 3,500,000 cases.

In 1989 Lytle and Stamper reported on 20 years of anesthesia experience with the almost 200 members of the Southern California Society of Oral and Maxillofacial Surgeons. The incidence of mortality was 1 death in every 633,000 anesthetics given.[96]

The trend in most offices is to provide sedation and local anesthesia for minor surgical procedures, with general anesthetics reserved for a small number of cases that specifically require it. In recent years, the administration of deep sedation, utilizing multiple drugs, has come to be regarded as the equivalent of general anesthesia where the patient has lost consciousness or cannot respond appropriately to question or command and is not in control of protective reflexes.

Allen indicates that Brevital appears to avoid the problems of complex cardiac dysrhythmias seen with induction of inhalation techniques, but there is usually a 40% to 50% increase in heart rate.[48] Other parameters studied show that Brevital and Pentothal without atropine comedication produced the least disturbance in blood pressure, total peripheral resistance, stroke volume, and cardiac output. Allen concludes that "out-patient anesthesia may indeed be demonstrated to be better than in-patient anesthesia."[48]

Campbell et al showed that overdosage and hypoxia were the two leading causes of morbidity and mortality leading to supraventricular tachyarrhythmias, which can decrease coronary blood flow by approximately 35%.[54] The addition of potent narcotics causes a significant decrease in PaO_2 (approximately 30 mm Hg) and an increase in $PaCO_2$—indicative of respiratory depression. On room air, hypoventilation occurs. Adding at least 30% oxygen and assisting ventilation readily restores the PaO_2 to normal range. Obese patients and those with anatomic abnormalities, for example, retrognathia, large tongue, and short neck, are especially at risk for airway obstruction, hypoventilation, and hypoxemia. Campbell et al recommend the routine use of at least 35% to 40% oxygen for deep sedation or general anesthesia cases.

VAGAL BLOCKING AGENTS

The routine use of anticholinergic drugs such as atropine prior to anesthesia with intravenous barbiturates has fallen from favor.[55] It has not been shown to materially affect the incidence of dysrhythmias encountered in outpatient general anesthesia situations and produces a marked fall in total peripheral resistance, particularly if venous return is compromised.[55]

Atropine and scopolamine (hyoscine) inhibit the muscarinic receptor sites in the postganglionic synapses of the parasympathetic and sympathetic nervous systems, which control the sweat glands.

Although the anticipated response to atropine is tachycardia, a biphasic action may show an early transient bradycardia. Atropine may also precipitate dysrhythmias, more often seen with small dosages. The incidence and severity of ventricular ectopic rhythms have been associated with painful or stressful stimulation by the surgical procedures.

Both vagal blocking drugs have also been used to dry secretions, nowadays of less concern with newer anesthetic agents (with the exception of ketamine). Scopolamine in equivalent doses to atropine is twice as potent a drying agent and lasts longer. Interestingly, atropine blocks mainly mucous cell secretions; the serous cells are less affected. It may also potentiate the problem of gastric regurgitation by decreasing the tone of the lower esophageal sphincter.

Central nervous system effects clearly differentiate between atropine and scopolamine. Atropine has mild sedative effects, whereas scopolamine produces pronounced sedation and often dissociation because its CNS activity is 10 times as potent as that of atropine.

The systemic use of atropine or scopolamine does not significantly affect intraocular pressure; these drugs may be used in patients with glaucoma.[56,57]

Atropine blocks sweat production and may interfere with temperature control, especially in children. Shutt and Bowes advise that the intramuscular use of atropine in the adult is inadequate and offers little or no vagal blockage while producing undesirable side affects.[56] Its intravenous use should be limited to specific indications such as countering the bradycardia induced by beta-blocking drugs or muscle relaxants.[52,55]

Glycopyrrolate (Robinul) has been recommended as a substitute for atropine.[58] It causes less tachycardia and better drying of secretions, although this latter effect lasts much longer than necessary, especially for ambulatory anesthesia cases. Glycopyrrolate does not cross the blood-brain barrier and hence produces no CNS effects.

Bourne advised that the amnesic effects of methohexital were achieved with the administration of as little as 0.5 mg/kg.[47] (For a 70-kg man this would mean just 35 mg!) He hastens to add that such a small dose would not obtund pain and would cause the patient to react to the stimulus and interfere with the operation, although he may not recall the reaction later. This effect undoubtedly explains the success of the "minimal incremental technique" of methohexital used for conservative dentistry and advocated by S. L. Drummond-Jackson[59] and his associates, particularly when the operative procedures are nonpainful. The use of local anesthesia to block impulses, plus the administration of minimal amounts of methohexital to effect sedation and amnesia, have made this method a very useful one. It must be emphasized that methohexital is considered a general anesthetic and is not meant for conscious sedation. The margin of difference between an awake patient and an unconscious patient is much too narrow with methohexital. Education and training in general anesthesia techniques are essential when methohexital is used.

For outpatient general anesthesia with methohexital, following a small test dose of 10 to 20 mg, the patient is slowly titrated to unconsciousness. A bite block is placed and the mouth is propped open prior to induction. The absence of the eyelid reflex serves as a helpful although not completely reliable guide to this light level of unconsciousness. This may occur within 30 to 40 seconds and is usually accompanied by a pronounced increase in heart rate when the medication "hits." Close monitoring of the patient's respirations and heart rate is maintained. Via an indwelling needle in the patient's vein, further increments of methohexital are given as needed. Again, the patient's reactions serve as the most reliable guide to the need for more drug, rather than any fixed idea of "appropriate dosage." The back of the mouth is packed off without interfering with the nasal and oropharyngeal airways. The packing is a 4 × 8 inch padded gauze screen and is changed as often as required to keep it reasonably dry and effective to catch any debris, saliva, or blood. The surgical assistant is key to the success of this technique and must maintain an active vigil to keep the oropharynx free of unwarranted material. Suctioning is important, as is the forward positioning of the tongue and jaw to avoid airway obstruction.

The anesthetist or anesthetic assistant of the surgical-anesthesia team[49] maintains the mandible in a forward position to avoid compromising the airway and monitors the pulse and respiration. Very short procedures (under 5 minutes) are usually done without any adjunctive nitrous oxide–oxygen nasal inhalation. Longer operations often benefit from additional supplementation with potent inhalation anesthetics such as halothane. Early awakening after methohexital is rapid, but this by no means indicates recovery. Studies show that recovery of psychomotor function after a short methohexital anesthesia takes more than 1 ½ hours,[58] and EEG changes are evident up to 12 hours later. This drug is only slowly broken down in the body but is rapidly redistributed with a resultant decline of its level in the brain after a very few minutes. Its redistribution into the muscle and fat stores of the body accounts for the slow recovery.

Techniques in intravenous anesthesia are continuously evolving. Many dentists are now using a small dose of diazepam or midazolam intravenously prior to the methohexital induction. Clinically, they serve to decrease the overall dose of methohexital required and produce a smoother anesthesia with no significant increase in recovery time.

The introduction of benzodiazepine antagonists (e.g., flumazenil) will materially change the practice of both conscious sedation and general anesthesia. This drug has been shown to effect a prompt reversal and awakening in patients who were comatose secondary to benzodiazepine overdosage.[60] The antagonist's effect lasted for 1 to 2 hours.

Propanidid, a eugenol derivative introduced in the United Kingdom for intravenous use in 1967, has fallen into disuse because of toxicity and adverse cardiovascular effects.

Etomidate is a new intravenous anesthetic belonging to the imidazole chemical group and chemically unrelated to any other hypnotic agent. The aqueous solution is unstable and loses potency within 24 hours. Given intravenously in dosage of 0.3 mg/kg, it causes sleep within one arm-brain circulation time. It is very rapidly broken down by esterase hydrolysis, but detectable amounts are found in the plasma up to 6 hours later. Injection is painful in smaller veins, and involuntary muscular movements, tremors, and hypertonia may follow. Like methohexital, it causes hiccuping and coughing. It appears to have minimal adverse cardiovascular effects and does not evoke a histamine release.[61]

Recovery is very rapid, taking approximately half the time when compared to thiopental but longer than methohexital.[62,63] There is also a higher incidence of nausea postoperatively. A more recent finding was that etomidate causes adrenal cortical suppression even after one bolus dose.[64] In a recent study comparing etomidate and methohexital, the carbon dioxide ventilatory response showed similar depressant effects on the medullary center for both drugs.[65] However, etomidate caused a stimulation of respiration (independent of carbon dioxide tension) and was recommended as the "logical choice for induction in cases where spontaneous ventilation is desired."[65]

Dissociative Anesthesia: Ketamine Hydrochloride (Ketalar)

The phenyl cyclohexidine group of compounds, notably ketamine hydrochloride, produces an altered state of consciousness that is quite distinct from that usually seen with conventional inhalational and intravenous anesthetics. Administered either intramuscularly or intravenously, ketamine rapidly produces profound analgesia and a cataleptic state in which the patient appears dissociated from the environment. The eyes remain open with a slow nystagmic gaze, and light and corneal reflexes persist intact. Electroencephalographic studies show excitatory activity in the thalamus and limbic systems, but the drug does not provoke seizure activity.[66] Vital functions are not depressed; in fact, cardiovascular function and respiration are well maintained. Although it is claimed that laryngeal and pharyngeal reflexes are not obtunded, a very high percentage of patients show laryngeal soiling, with an increase in salivary and tracheobronchial secretions.

When used in the original dosage recommended by the manufacturer (i.e., 5 mg/lb intramuscularly for children and 1 mg/lb intravenously for adults), a very high incidence of prolonged, disturbed recovery, with vomiting (40% to 60%) and psychomimetic reactions, occurred. Becsey et al utilized droperidol to diminish these adverse affects.[67] However, droperidol is a long-acting agent and not suitable for ambulatory use. McLaughlin and Corcoran expressed "second thoughts" on the use of ketamine, based on their experience with adverse effects such as hypertension, vomiting, profuse salivation, laryngospasm, respiratory obstruction, and frightening hallucinatory episodes on emergence from anesthesia.[68]

For outpatient anesthesia, experience has served to reduce the original dosage recommended and to limit its use to young children. Greenfield advised the following be administered—for children under 50 lb: 0.5 to 0.75 mg/lb; 50 to 100 lb: 0.75 to 1.0 mg/lb; over 100 lb: 1.0 to 1.5 mg/lb.[69] These dosages represent approximately 10% of the original recommendation.

When ketamine is given to children, there is a dissociative state achieved within 4 minutes after intramuscular injection. When the drug is given intravenously, this state is achieved within 30 seconds. The drug stimulates salivary secretions, often with attendant laryngeal spasm possible. This has been largely overcome by the use of scopolamine or atropine give intramuscularly 15 to 20 minutes before ketamine is used, or glycopyrrolate 0.005 mg/kg IV 5 to 10 minutes prior to induction.

With these smaller doses recovery times are not unduly prolonged. Greenfield reports that almost all patients recovered within 30 minutes; the majority recovered in less than 15 minutes.[69] He also found a less profound dissociation that even enabled conversation with the older patients. Yet anterograde amnesia postoperatively was complete. Where the analgesia obtained was inadequate, he used 50% nitrous oxide–oxygen supplementation or local anesthesia. There were no instances of vomiting or adverse psychomotor reactions reported in over 700 patients so managed.

Low-dose ketamine hydrochloride (0.5 mg/kg) intravenously combined with diazepam (0.15 mg/kg) did not prolong recovery and served to reduce untoward emergence reactions. Benzodiazepines (e.g., diazepam and midazolam) are highly effective in preventing marked cardiovascular responses and unpleasant emergence reactions.[66] An innovation by Nagashima is the administration of ketamine hydrochloride 2.5 to 4.0 mg/kg together with hyaluronidase (Wydase) 0.2 ml (30 units) intramuscularly.[70] This leads to a more rapid onset of anesthesia (2 to 3 minutes) and a shorter duration, with recoveries between 40 and 60 minutes. It has been used primarily in children and has shown no untoward effects. It has also helped to diminish or eliminate some of the CNS excitatory effects.[71]

Contraindications to the use of ketamine include patients with significant cardiovascular disease, such as poorly controlled hypertension, congestive heart failure, intracranial, thoracic, or abdominal aneurysm, and unstable angina. Procedures involving pharynx, larynx, or trachea are considered to be relative contraindications.[65]

For the present, ketamine for the outpatient has found a limited place and is more often used for short procedures in young children. Hopefully it portends the coming of other related agents that can be used to great advantage once the disturbing side effects are eliminated.

Propofol (Diprivan)

Propofol is a newly introduced intravenous hypnotic agent intended for induction and maintenance of short-term anesthesia. Chemically it is 2,6-Di-isopropylphenol. It is formulated as an oily emulsion with a pH of 7.0 to 8.5 and supplied in 20-ml ampules of 10 mg/ml. Intravenous injection of propofol produces hypnosis within 40 seconds with minimal excitation. Pharmacokinetically, an IV bolus dose shows a rapid-phase half-life of less than 10 minutes and a slower phase of up to 1 hour. Its elimination requires 5 to 12 hours. Clinically, recovery from a single bolus dose of 2.0 to 2.5 mg/kg occurs within minutes. Other drugs that cause CNS depression serve to increase the CNS depression induced by propofol.

Hemodynamically, hypotension occurs frequently on induction, with minimal change in heart rate or cardiac output. Assisted ventilation or premedication with a potent opioid (e.g., fentanyl) further decreases cardiac output.

Induction with propofol is also frequently associated with apnea, which may be prolonged (i.e., >30 sec in 35% of patients). An increase in carbon dioxide tension is associated with this depression of respiration.

This anesthetic is not recommended for use during pregnancy, for nursing mothers, or for pediatric patients. Caution is also advised for patients with increased intracranial pressure or impaired cerebral circulation, as well as for elderly or debilitated patients.

Transient local pain on administration may occur, but phlebothrombosis is very rare. Perivascular or inadvertent intra-arterial injection has been reported to cause no major sequelae.

Dosage is individualized, with healthy adults likely to require 2.0 to 2.5 mg/kg for inductions. Intermittently, increments of 25 mg to 50 mg are given as needed. One of the major advantages of propofol is the rapidity of recovery compared with other intravenous anesthetics.

The acceptance of propofol into dental anesthesiology practice has been slow. This may reflect a move away from general anesthesia and toward conscious sedation management of patients in the office setting.

Monitoring

Anesthesia monitoring has significantly advanced over the past decade, largely because of innovations in electronic technology. For the short office anesthetic case, close monitoring is still readily and reliably accomplished by the use of either a precordial or suprastenal stethoscope connected to a molded earpiece (Fig. 8-1). Breathing and heart sounds are monitored

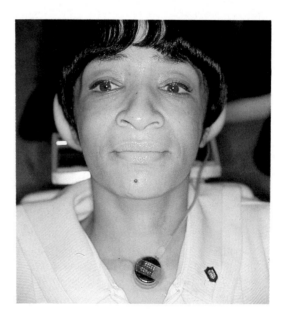

Fig. 8-1. Suprasternal stethoscope aids in monitoring respiration and transmitted heart sounds.

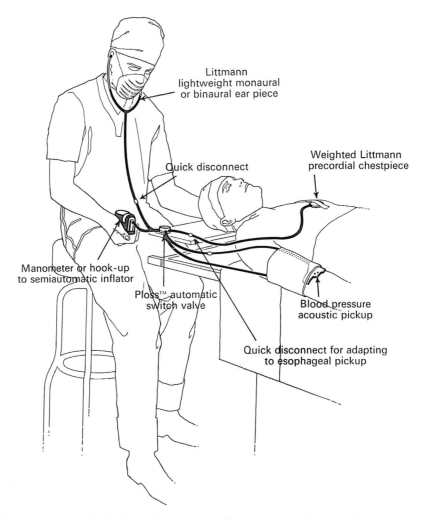

Littmann
lightweight monaural
or binaural ear piece

Quick disconnect

Weighted Littmann
precordial chestpiece

Manometer or hook-up
to semiautomatic inflator

Ploss™ automatic
switch valve

Blood pressure
acoustic pickup

Quick disconnect for adapting
to esophageal pickup

Fig. 8-2. Ploss valve for monitoring blood pressure and heart sounds. (Courtesy 3M Co.)

aurally by the position of the suprasternal stethoscope head. By the use of a Ploss* automatic switch valve, both the blood pressure and the heart sounds may be readily detected (Fig. 8-2). In our experience these measures are reliable and more often freer of artifacts than electronic finger or ear pulse monitors or even an ECG apparatus. For most short procedures in healthy patients, the ECG may be an unnecessary encumbrance.

Noninvasive monitoring is preferred, especially in the outpatient or office setting. An amplified stethoscope head (CardioSonic*), which helps to overcome extraneous room noises and enhances breath and heart sounds is available.

One of the newly "required" and most promising electronic monitoring aids is the pulse oximeter. This instrument, attached to the finger, provides continuous information on the oxygen saturation at the peak of the pulse wave

---

*3M Co., St. Paul, Minn.

*SRS Co., Napa, Calif.

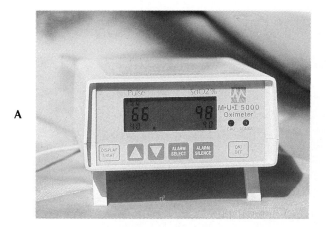

A

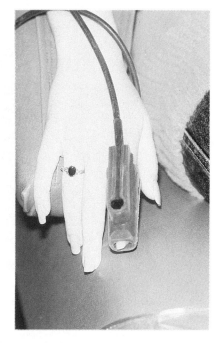

B

Fig. 8-3. **A,** Pulse oximeter monitors oxygen saturation and also provides heart beat signals. **B,** Noninvasive finger adaptor for pulse oximeter.

(Fig. 8-3). Unlike the transcutaneous oxygen monitoring system, it does not require preheating or an extended time to achieve a steady state and recalibration. Pulse oximetry works by positioning a pulsating arterial vascular bed between a two-wavelength light source and a detector. The vascular bed, by expanding and relaxing in plethysmographic fashion, creates a change in the length of the light's path that modifies the amount of light detected, producing a typical plethysmographic wave form and providing beat-to-beat calculation of arterial oxygen saturation.[72]

In a study conducted at Montefiore Medical Center, a pulse oximeter (Minolta/Marquest Finger Oximeter*) was compared with arterial blood samples taken from an indwelling arterial line during major hospital anesthesia cases. Excellent correlation between the two methods was obtained over a wide range (55% to 100%)

of oxyhemoglobin concentrations. Similar results were reported by Swerdlow and Stern.[73] It is important to appreciate that the hazards of hypoxia often herald the coming of cardiac dysrhythmias. Monitoring of respiration is crude—clinically it depends on counting the rate of respiration and estimating changes in tidal volumes or the depth of respiration by observing movements of the chest wall. It becomes difficult to assess whether hypoxia is present. Only several minutes later does the electrical activity of the heart become erratic.

The pulse oximeter can be highly recommended as a noninvasive monitor of both respiration and heart rate. It would be equally appropriate for use even in "sedation cases," particularly when multiple drugs are used and a deeper level of sedation is coupled with interference with the airway. This poses a hazard that is difficult to recognize, one that would be readily detected by a pulse oximeter. The instrument has alarm settings that alert the anesthetist just as soon as the low saturation barrier is

---

*Minolta/Marquest Co., Englewood, Colo.

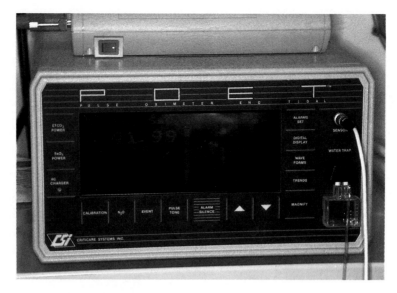

Fig. 8-4. Capnograph measuring end-tidal carbon dioxide.

breached. The pulse oximeter is also used routinely now in hospital recovery rooms, where early warning of impending hypoxia is equally critical.

Monitoring of end-tidal carbon dioxide has not only become readily available based on technologic advances but has even been mandated by certain state regulations. It certainly provides valuable information for general anesthesia cases involving endotracheal intubation. Noninvasive capnography may also be helpful for nonintubated cases. Capnographs* with and without printers are available that record CO_2 tension, respiratory rate, and wave forms, and provide alarm systems to identify some of the earliest adverse physiologic changes (Fig. 8-4).

Postanesthesia monitoring for the ambulatory patient in the recovery room has been well detailed by Delo, Mulkey, and Davis.[74] They have incorporated closed-circuit television monitors into their recovery area to supervise their patients. Generally, ambulatory patients are awake and in control of their reflexes before being transferred to the recovery area. Most patients walk, with assistance, to the recovery room, which is equipped with auxiliary suction and oxygen.

Neurophysiologic Effects of Anesthetics

Electroencephalographic studies show that barbiturates initiate rapid, large waves that begin in the frontal brain areas and progress caudally.[75] They first excite cortical neurons in areas of the mesencephalic reticular formation.[76] Deepening anesthesia is associated with the appearance of spindle-shaped bursts that coincide with unconsciousness. Further deepening leads to large polymorphic waves, at which point the patient tolerates skin incision. Beyond this point the EEG shows periods of suppression that alternate with bursts of high-frequency waves. Suppressions caused by barbiturates become prolonged as concentration rises and the mesencephalic reticular formation undergoes progressive depression.[76] When sensory-evoked responses are measured, barbiturates clearly do not reduce these potentials, representing response to external stimuli. In fact, there is enhancement of sensory-evoked potentials firing the early phase of barbiturate anesthesia. Clin-

---

*Microspan 8090 Capnograph Monitor, Bichom Monitors Unlimited, Dayton, Ohio.

ically this may explain the "antianalgesic" effect of barbiturates.

Concentrations of nitrous oxide as high as 30% rarely alter the EEG, although psychologic functions are disturbed. Higher concentrations serve to cause progressive loss of alpha rhythm, which coincides with the development of unconsciousness. At higher concentrations, fast, irregular, low waves appear but slowing and suppression do not. The latter's absence indicates the lack of potency of nitrous oxide at atmospheric pressures. Only concentrations that produce unconsciousness caused a decrease in specific somatic-evoked potentials.[75] This corroborates our clinical impression that true analgesia does not occur with nitrous oxide unless the patient is rendered unconscious. In the conscious patient receiving nitrous oxide–oxygen sedation, psychologic alterations are primarily responsible for the decrease in reaction to painful and anxiety-provoking situations. Zuniga has demonstrated release of beta-endorphins in rats given higher concentrations (60% to 80%) of nitrous oxide.[77]

As with nitrous oxide, studies of methoxyflurane also show that concentrations that do not produce unconsciousness leave somatic potentials intact. This was borne out by Goldstein, Dragon, and Cobb (noted earlier) in their clinical study of analgesia in conscious patients receiving methoxyflurane.[42]

Enflurane induces rapid EEG activity early, which coincides with unconsciousness. Increased concentrations lead to larger waves that then turn into slower frequencies and smaller waves. Just as these dominate the EEG pattern, dramatic epileptoid bursts appear. These may contain the spike and dome complexes, indicative of CNS irritability.

Halothane-oxygen alone rapidly produces an increased frequency of higher waves that then slow at higher concentrations and may produce suppressions. When nitrous oxide is added the EEG pattern is changed and noxious stimuli can disrupt lower rhythmic waves. Analgesia coincides with the development of smaller waves and a slower EEG than when higher concentrations of halothane are used

alone. Neuroleptanalgesia as defined by Foldes is a "state of central nervous system depression with tranquilization and intense analgesia produced without use of barbiturate or volatile agents."[78] Ketamine hydrochloride, an agent that produces a new and different dissociative state of the CNS, has been associated with EEG changes, suggesting excitability of the brain and seizure activity.[79]

Hospital Inpatient Anesthesia

In general, anesthesia for the hospitalized patient undergoing dental and oral surgical treatment is not remarkably different from that given for other surgical procedures. However, the hospital anesthesiologist is often confronted by a sick patient who has been identified as unsuitable for office ambulatory anesthesia. In addition, the oral surgeon will usually hospitalize patients who are major surgical problems, for example, patients requiring fracture reductions as well as other extensive corrective and reconstructive oral surgery. The availability of special hospital services and consultations makes admission to the hospital mandatory for these special patients.

Hospital anesthesia for dentistry usually involves a more formal medical evaluation of the patient, which consists of a physical examination and laboratory tests such as hematocrit or hemoglobin determination and urinalysis as a basic minimum. Most hospitals also require an evaluation of the roentgenogram of the chest and an ECG for the adult patient. Because hospitalized dental patients constitute a special group of patients who are at greater risk, these extensive preoperative evaluations are justified. They do create a significant physical and economic burden for the patient and should not be considered a viable alternative to office anesthesia for most healthy patients who require anesthesia for dental treatment.

Same day admission of patients for elective procedures is now common. Patients usually fast from before midnight to the morning of the scheduled surgery. If the operation is planned for later in the day, many hospitals will allow an early breakfast of clear liquids. A period of 6 to

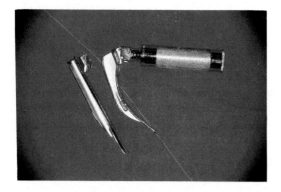

Fig. 8-5. Laryngoscope with both straight and curved blades available.

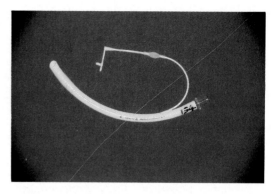

Fig. 8-6. Endotracheal tube with expansile balloon attached to ensure better seal of the pharynx.

8 hours of fasting is the common rule for elective surgical cases. The anesthesiologist visits the patient the evening before surgery, reviews the patient's history and laboratory data, and prescribes pre-operative medication. A hypnotic agent is often prescribed to encourage relaxation and sleep the night before surgery. Most anesthesiologists will also prescribe medication to be injected intramuscularly when the nurse receives word from the operating room personnel that the patient is "on call."

In the past a hypnotic agent such as pentobarbital sodium, a narcotic such as meperidine hydrochloride, and an anticholinergic drug such as atropine or scopolamine were administered 1 hour before scheduled surgery. Many substitutions are used: Benadryl, Vistaril, Phenergan, etc, may be used instead of Nembutal. Many anesthesiologists prefer not to prescribe a narcotic agent because the patient is not in pain, and sedation is more readily accomplished by barbiturates or tranquilizers without the attendant risk of respiratory depression resulting from the narcotic.

In the induction room or the operating room, anesthesia is usually preceded by the initiation of an intravenous drip with saline solution or 5% dextrose and water. If there is need for blood transfusion, nothing smaller than an 18-gauge needle is used. During the preparatory period, a blood pressure cuff is applied, a precordial stethoscope and ECG leads are taped to the chest, a pulse oximeter is attached to a finger, and baseline data are obtained. The nostrils and larynx are sprayed with a topical anesthetic or a vasoconstrictor (e.g., cocaine 4% to 10%).

For most adults, induction is with an intravenous injection of thiopental sodium followed by a period where a face mask is positioned and oxygen administered. A further increment of thiopental is then followed by an intravenous injection of succinylcholine—a potent short-acting muscle relaxant. Its effects are soon seen as fasciculation of the muscles of the chest, neck, and face. The mouth is then easily opened, a laryngoscope (Fig. 8-5) is inserted into the oropharynx, and a nasoendotracheal tube is guided through the abducted, paralyzed vocal cords by aid of Magill forceps. Once the tube is through the cords, it is advanced into the trachea to just above the branching of the right mainstem bronchus. The tube is connected to the anesthesia machine, and the anesthetist "bags" or ventilates the patient with oxygen. Because the patient is still paralyzed and cannot yet breathe on his or her own, he or she must be manually ventilated until the effect of the succinylcholine wears off. At this time, one checks to make sure that both sides of the chest rise with compression of the reservoir bag, to ascertain that the endotracheal tube has not been pushed too far and has come to rest in the right mainstem bronchus and can inflate only the right lung. The use of a capnograph to measure

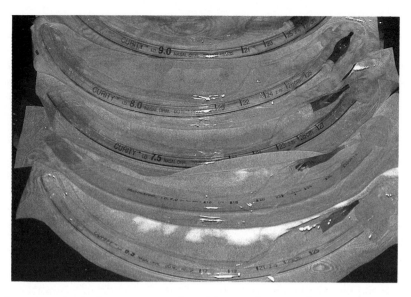

Fig. 8-7. Sterile endotracheal tubes are now packaged for one-time use. They come in a range of sizes to fit different-sized children and adults.

end-tidal carbon dioxide is now routine and ensures the proper tube position.

Most endotracheal tubes (Figs. 8-6 & 8-7) now also bear a small collapsible balloon on their outer surface, which is expanded with air to form a cuff and fill the hypopharynx around the tube. This ensures a better fit with less leakage of gases and prevents extraneous blood and debris from the oral cavity from entering the trachea. Once the tube is secured, the anesthesia may proceed by a variety of methods, depending upon the preference of the anesthetist, the anticipated duration of the surgery, and the medical status of the patient. Inhalational techniques using nitrous oxide, and halothane or enflurane, or isoflurane are commonly used. Shorter procedures may allow the anesthetist to continue to use thiopental intermittently if jaw relaxation is not difficult to maintain and if the patient is responding well to small doses of the drug. Arbitrarily most anesthetists will not want to give more than 1.0 to 1.5 g of thiopental. Some anesthetists will initate an IV drip of succinylcholine to paralyze the patient and maintain analgesia with 70% nitrous oxide with controlled ventilation. Others use a technique that

has been called *neuroleptanesthesia*. This may be achieved by the use of a potent tranquilizing agent such as droperidol (Inapsine) and a narcotic, either fentanyl citrate (Sublimaze), alftentanil,[80] or meperidine. The advantage of this latter technique is due to the availability of a highly effective and specific narcotic antagonist, naloxone hydrochloride (Narcan). At the end of surgery the anesthetist administers the antagonist, which effectively reverses all the narcotic's side effects, including the respiratory depression. Before the narcotic is reversed the patient will often require assisted ventilation.

Children are usually managed with an inhalational agent both for induction and maintenance of anesthesia. For very young children an oral endotracheal tube is preferred, to avoid nasal and adenoidal damage and bleeding. A larger-diameter tube can be used, which facilitates better ventilation. Young children are also managed with the use of ketamine (previously discussed in the section on ambulatory anesthesia).

Postoperatively, patients are watched over carefully in their hospital recovery room, where frequent checks are made of their vital signs.

The use of a pulse oximeter is quite common. Intravenous fluids are administered, and patients are returned to their own rooms when awake and stable. Endotracheal anesthesia is not without its problems. In the young, the irritant effect of the tube in the larynx promotes edema, which may produce respiratory stridor and, in severe cases, even respiratory obstruction. A cool-mist tent is used for recovering youngsters, and even adults benefit from a cool-mist mask while in the recovery room. If the intubation has been particularly traumatic or if the child's head has been moved from side to side during the operation, causing further laryngeal trauma from the endotracheal tube, a corticosteroid such as dexamethasone (Decadron) is given prophylactically to reduce the inflammatory response and the edema. Occasionally, trauma from the tube in the nose may initiate active bleeding, which on occasion requires a posterior nasal pack to arrest. Generally, patients compain of a sore throat on the day following surgery and may also complain of the numerous aches and pains they feel in their chest, abdomen, and back. These pains are muscular and related to the intense fasciculation induced by the succinylcholine. Reassurance as to their cause, a mild analgesic, and a hot bath will lead to rapid improvement. The period of apnea produced by the succinylcholine is a tense time for the anesthetist to locate the larynx, visualize the vocal cords, and pass the tube. In haste the anesthetist may incorrectly use the maxillary anterior teeth as a fulcrum for the laryngoscope and either fracture or sublux these teeth. Care and experience are necessary to use the laryngoscope properly and avoid damage.

Occasionally it becomes necessary to intubate a patient blindly—without the use of a laryngoscope (e.g., for the patient who has an ankylosis of the jaw and cannot open his or her mouth even after the muscles are paralyzed). Patients with severe mandibular retrognathia are also very difficult to intubate, as are patients with cervical spine injuries who cannot be manipulated. Finally, there is a time when patients are intubated while awake. This has been used in the previously mentioned cases and also when emergency surgery is required and the patient has eaten recently. Here the techniques involve topical anesthetization of the larynx or the administration of a transtracheal injection of local anesthesia prior to passing the tube. If the patient vomits, he or she is still awake and can cough and hopefully avoid aspiration of gastric contents. In some difficult-to-intubate cases, a fiberoptic bronchoscope is threaded down the lumen of the endotracheal tube, enabling one to visualize the cords, advance the endotracheal tube, and pull out the bronchoscope probe once the tube has entered the trachea.

Gastric Acid Aspiration

Vomiting and aspiration of gastric contents contribute to significant anesthetic morbidity and mortality. The prophylactic use of an antacid has been advocated to increase gastric pH and minimize its corrosive effect if aspirated into the lung. More recently, the use of preoperative histamine (H_2) antagonist drugs such as cimetidine (Tagamet) or ranitidine hydrochloride (Zantac) has been strongly advocated.[81] In children, a 0.1 to 0.3 mg/kg dose of cimetidine given between 1 and 4 hours before anesthesia significantly reduced both the volume and acidity of gastric fluid.[82] For emergency surgery and anesthesia, a nasogastric tube is passed, the stomach is evacuated, and 30 ml of 0.3 M sodium citrate is instilled.[85] The prophylactic use of cimetidine has also been advocated for ambulatory, nonpremedicated, anxious children who undergo anesthetic induction by mask and are at increased risk for vomiting and aspiration during general anesthesia.[83]

Malignant Hyperthermia

This potentially fatal syndrome is seen in a small percentage of the population exposed to a variety of anesthetic agents, such as muscle relaxants, inhalation and intravenous general anesthetic agents, atropine, and even phenothiazines, for example, promethazine (Phenergan). In its full-blown form it is characterized by muscle rigidity, tachycardia, and tachyarrhythmias, a rapidly rising temperature, acidosis secondary to increased metabolic breakdown, and hypercapnia. The plasma shows elevated creatine phosphokinase (CPK) related to muscle catabolism. If the condition is untreated, there is a very high mortality rate. Dantrolene sodium is advocated and available before starting anesthesia and continuing intravenously at a dosage of 2.5 mg/kg should a hyperthermic episode develop.[84] Dantrolene acts as a skeletal muscle relaxant by dissociating excitation-contraction coupling and by inhibition of calcium ion release from the cell's sarcoplasmic reticulum. It has no appreciable effect on cardiac or smooth muscle.[84] The disease is believed to be inherited as an autosomal dominant with variable expression and an incidence of 1:15,000 to 1:50,000.

Masseter spasm, often cited as an early indicator of the syndrome, was studied in relation to succinylcholine administration.[85] Of all children studied, 1% showed masseter spasm when exposed to succinylcholine/halothane anesthesia, with significant elevations in CPK. However, none of the children progressed to classic malignant hyperthermia once the halothane was withdrawn or the case was aborted. Muscle biopsies from 12 of the 15 children were all positive for malignant hyperthermia susceptibility. The authors of this study advise that the masseter spasm should not be dismissed as a benign event.[85]

Larach and Rosenberg reported on anesthetic responses in 15 malignant hyperthermia-susceptible children managed for muscle biopsy with thiopental, nitrous oxide–oxygen, pancuronium, and fentanyl.[86] Total body rigidity was predictive of positive muscle biospy. Masseter rigidity was found in 73% of positive muscle biopsy and 50% of negative muscle biopsy cases.

A number of diseases have been associated with malignant hyperthermia (e.g., myopathies), such as the myopathies associated with osteogenesis imperfecta and Duchenne's dystrophy.[87]

It is prudent to obtain a temperature baseline on each patient before anesthesia and to maintain a temperature probe in place for all but the shortest of anesthesia cases.

Mortality Associated with Anesthesia

Anesthesiology departments continually review their experiences on a regular basis, particularly with regard to fatalities associated with anesthesia. In many hospitals a death report for each patient who dies within 7 days of operation is completed and reviewed. Marx, Mateo, and Orkin reviewed over 34,000 anesthesia cases and found that 645 patients had died within this postoperative period.[88] The two prime determinants of mortality were: (1) the physical status of the patient and (2) the judgment and skill of the anesthesiologist. The site of surgery was also a prominent determinant of outcome, with the heart, great vessels, and brain leading the list. The incidence of death was lowest between the ages of 1 and 30 years. The death rate was highest on the day of operation and the first postoperative day and declined progressively thereafter. The overall mortality rate of 1.82% was favorably compared with the National Halothane Study rate of 1.93% for all anesthetics.

Other studies, such as the Baltimore Anesthesia Committee's "Factors in Geriatric Anesthesia Mortality,"[89] also emphasize the significance of physical status and aging in relation to higher mortality. For patients over 65 years of age the mortality rate was almost five times that experienced by younger patients.

Lewin et al showed a direct relationship between anesthetic mortality in the aged and duration of anesthesia.[90] They experienced a zero mortality rate for cases anesthetized for less than 2 hours; 21% for cases anesthetized for 2 to 4 hours; 71% for cases anesthetized for more than 4 hours; and 80% for cases anesthetized for over 6 hours.

One of the principal direct causes of death in the Baltimore survey[89] was aspiration of vomitus; others were neuromuscular depression and cardiovascular collapse. Aspiration had been cited in other reports as the leading cause of death in pediatric and obstetric anesthesia and anesthesia of the traumatized patient.[91]

Mauney, Ebert, and Sabiston established an important relationship between intraoperative hypotension and subsequent myocardial infarction.[92] In this study 16 of the 30 patients who sustained myocardial damage succumbed. The presence of ischemic heart disease is known to significantly affect the outcome of anesthesia and surgery. Patients with recent myocardial infarctions show a very high mortality when subjected to anesthesia. The incidence is as high as 77% initially and then decreases over the next 6 months to 1 year. However, even after the first year the risk of mortality and postoperative myocardial infarction is still 10 times higher than in patients without a history of previous myocardial disease.[93] Anesthesia for elective dental treatment is usually avoided entirely, if possible. An alternative is to offer the patient intravenous (conscious) sedation plus local anesthesia.

In a recent prospective study of the likelihood of serious complication developing in the operating room and/or in the recovery room, Vaughan et al were able to predict complications based on selected preoperative and intraoperative conditions. These included patients with initial physical status of ASA III, major organ system disease, multiple preoperative and antibiotic therapy, abdominal incision, and prolonged operative procedures.[94]

Other major sources of anesthetic morbidity and mortality relate to improper intubation of the trachea, hypovolemia, drug overdosage, unrecognized hypotension, and various mechanical equipment failures. Wilson cites a recent British study of anesthetic mortality as 1:10,000 cases.[95] He indicates that this statistic has unfortunately not shown improvement over the past decade.

One cannot compare statistics on outpatient versus inpatient anesthesia—it is like comparing apples and oranges. Both are spherical and both are fruits, but there the analogy ends. However, in both types of management the mortality should be extremely low, and indeed it is. With proper preanesthetic evaluation of the patient, knowledgeable selection of the most appropriate anesthetic agents, and skill in the administration and monitoring of the case, mortality approaches zero. The well trained anesthetist is prepared to anticipate and avoid potential problems and is also ready to provide any emergency and resuscitative care.

Summary

General anesthesia for dental and oral surgical treatment can be realistically divided into two major categories—ambulatory (outpatient or office) and hospital (inpatient). Particularly in the area of ambulatory general anesthesia, dentistry has achieved an enviable record of safe, effective, and economical operations. Many of the innovations developed by the well-trained dentist and oral surgeon in the management of generally healthy office patients are well recognized and becoming more widely practiced by medical anesthesiologists for short procedures in an outpatient or surgicenter setting. Specifically, these techniques avoid heavy premedication, deep general anesthesia, tracheal intubation, and prolonged recovery. They provide for cases requiring anesthesia of relatively short duration, varying from 1 minute to 30 minutes. This is usually accomplished with the administration of intravenous methohexital for induction and inhalational agents such as nitrous oxide, and halothane. Propofol (Diprivan), which was recently introduced as an appropriate alternative to methohexital for short procedures, is becoming increasingly popular. The management of young children is generally done with halothane or other inhalational agents.

Because of the exaggerated concern about the relationship of hepatitis to the use of halothane, additional caution has been introduced and other agents are being recommended, for example, enflurane and isoflurane. It would be unfortunate if halothane were to be relegated to only occasional use, because it has proven to be a remarkably safe and effective agent. This dilemma is reviewed at length earlier in this chapter. Recent data relating to the neurophysiologic effects of anesthetics are presented, and the modifications in the use of ketamine for ambulatory anesthesia are discussed.

"Hospital" anesthesia for dental treatment differs very little from that given for other surgical procedures. It relies on routine premedication, tracheal intubation with muscle relaxants, and slower recovery under hospital supervision. It requires extensive preoperative medical evaluation, including chest radiographs, ECGs, and other laboratory tests, in addition to a physical examination. This is justified because most hospitalized general anesthesia patients are usually poorer risks or require major treatment for traumatic injuries or reconstructive surgery.

There are obvious attendant risks associated with general anesthesia. Serious problems relate to aspiration of vomitus and to the physical status of the patient, in addition to the skill and competence of the anesthetist. Advanced patient age, myocardial disease, and prolonged anesthesia all negatively influence the outcome.

Mortality associated with outpatient and inpatient anesthesia for dentistry and oral surgery cannot be readily compared. In most instances there are important differences with regard to physical status of the patient, extent of surgery, and anesthetic techniques.

References

1. Thompson EC: Letter to the editor, *J Mo Dent Assoc* 15:4, 1935.
2. Hubbell AO, Royer QR: *A method of outpatient general anesthesia for the oral surgical patient.* In Jorgensen NB et al, editors: *Sedation, local and general anesthesia in dentistry, 2,* Philadelphia, 1972, Lea & Febiger.
3. Cohen DD, Dillon JB: Anesthesia for outpatient surgery, *J Am Med Assoc* 196:1114-1116, 1966.
4. Ahlgren EW: Pediatric outpatient anesthesia—a four-year review, *Am J Dis Child* 126:36-38, 1973.
5. Lortie E: Th use of halothane in dental anesthesia, *J Can Dent Assoc* 27:77, 1961.
6. Kamen S: Dentistry for mentally retarded children, *NY State Dent J* 27:79, 1961.
7. Raventos J: The action of fluothane—a new volatile anesthetic, *Br J Pharmacol* 11:394, 1956.
8. Johnson M: The human cardiovascular response to fluothane anaesthesia, *Br J Anaesth* 28:392, 1956.
9. Trieger N: Fluothane anesthesia for ambulatory oral surgery patients, *Oral Surg Oral Med Oral Pathol* 16(1):31-34.
10. Trieger N: Halothane anesthesia for oral surgery patients treated in the office, *J Oral Surg* 23:595-599, 1965.
11. Dripps RD, Eckenhoff JE, Vandam LD: *Introduction to anesthesia—the principles of safe practice,* ed 6, Philadelphia, 1982, WB Saunders.
12. Fukunaga AF, Epstein RM: Sympathetic excitation duration nitrous oxide-halothane anesthesia in the cat, *Anesthesiology* 39(1):23-35, 1973.
13. Matteo RS, Katz RL, Papper EM: The injection of epinephrine during general anesthesia with halogenated hydrocarbons and cyclopropane in man, *Anesthesiology* 24:327, 1963.
14. Ngai SH, Mark LC, Papper MD: Pharmacologic and physiologic aspects of anesthesiology, *N Engl J Med* 282(10):541-556, 1970.
15. Karl HW, et al: Epinephrine-halothane interaction in children, *Anesthesiology* 58:142-145, 1983.
16. Subcommittee on the National Halothane Study of the Committee on Anesthesia, National Academy of Sciences: National Research Council Summary of the National Halothane Study, *J Am Med Assoc* 197:755-788, 1966.
17. Fisher DM et al: Comparison of enflurane, halothane, and isoflurane for outpatient pediatric anesthesia, *Anesthesiology* 61(3a):A427, 1984.
18. Strumin L, Simpson BR: Halothane in Britain today, *Br J Anaesth* 44: 919-924, 1972.
19. Little DM: *Effects of halothane on hepatic function.* In Greene NM, editor: *Halothane,* Philadelphia, 1968, FA Davis.
20. Klatskin G, Kimberg DV: Recurrent hepatitis attributable to halothane sensitization in an anesthetist, *N Engl J Med* 280:515-522, 1969.
21. Klion FM, Schaffner F, Popper H: Hepatitis after exposure to halothane, *Ann Intern Med* 71(3):467-477, 1969.
22. Carney FMT, Van Dyke RA: Halothane hepatitis: a critical review, *Anesth Analg* 51(1): 135:160, 1972.
23. Dykes MHM, Gilbert JP, McPeek B: Halothane in the United States, *Br J Anaesth* 44:925-934, 1972.
24. Lomanto C, Howland WS: Problems in diagnosing halothane hepatitis, *J Am Med Assoc* 214:1257-1261, 1970.
25. Bruce DL: What is a "safe" interval between halothane exposures, *J Am Med Assoc* 221(10): 1140-1142, 1972.
26. Trey C et al: Fulminant hepatic failures, presumable contribution of halothane, *N Engl J Med* 279:798-801, 1968.

27. Simpson BR, Strumin L, Walton B: The halothane dilemma: a case for the defense, *Br Med J* 4:96-100, 1971.

28. Davies GE, Holmes JE: Drug-induced immunological effects on the liver, *Br J Anaesth* 44:941, 1972.

29. Paronetto F, Popper H: Lymphocyte stimulation induced by halothane in patients with hepatitis following exposure to halothane, *N Engl J Med* 283:277-280, 1970.

30. Vergani D et al: Antibodies to the surface of halothane-altered rabbit hepatocytes in patients with severe halothane-associated hepatitis, *N Engl J Med* 303(2):66-71, 1980.

31. Dienstag JL: Halothane hepatitis—allergy or idiosyncrasy? *N Engl J Med* 303(2):102-103, 1980.

32. Ross WT Jr: Plasma fluoride concentration during halogenated anesthetic administration with normoxia and hypoxia, *Anesthesiology* V57(3):A217, 1982.

33. Shingu K et al: Effect of oxygen concentration on anesthetic-induced hepatic injury in rats, *Anesthesiology* V57(3):A219, 1982.

34. Solosko D, Frissell M, Smith RB: 111 halothane anesthesias in a pediatric patient: a case report, *Anesth Analg* 51(5):706-709, 1972.

35. Lewis RB, Blair M: Halothane hepatitis in a young child, *Br J Anaesth* 54:349-354, 1982.

36. Stewart G, McGovern J: Penicillin allergy: clinical and immunologic aspects (II), Springfield, Ill, 1970, Charles C Thomas.

37. Lebowitz M, Blitt CD, Dillon JB: Clinical investigations of compound 347 (Ethrane), *Anesth Analg* 49:1-10, 1970.

38. Dobkin AB et al: Ethrane (compound 347) anesthesia: a clinical and laboratory review of 700 cases, *Anesth Analg* 48(3):477-494, 1969.

39. Marshall BE et al: Some pulmonary and cardiovascular effects of enflurane (Ethrane) anesthesia with varying $PaCO_2$ in man, *Br J Anaesth* 43:996-1002, 1971.

40. Trieger N, Lasner J: Enflurane ambulatory anesthesia: recovery compared to intravenous anesthesia, *Anesth Prog* 22:1, 1975.

41. Hetrick WD, Wolfson B, Garcia DA: Renal responses to "light" methoxyflurance anesthesia, *Anesthesiology* 38(1):30-39, 1973.

42. Goldstein IC, Dragon AI, Cobb S: Inhalation analgesia by nasal cannula and nasal hood: an alternative to narcotics? *Anesth Prog* 15(10):289-294, 1968.

43. Allen GD: *Dental anesthesia and analgesia,* Baltimore, 1984, William & Wilkins Co.

44. Linde HW, Dykes MHM: Evaluation of a general anesthetic—Isoflurane, *J Am Med Assoc* 245(2):2335-2336, 1981.

45. Eger EI, II. *Uptake and distribution of inhaled anesthetics.* In Miller D, editor: *Anesthesia,* New York, 1981, Churchill Livingstone.

46. Gold MI, Durate I, Muravchick S: Arterial oxygenation in conscious patients after five minutes and after 30 seconds of oxygen breathing, *Anesth Anal* 60:316-316, 1981.

47. Bourne JG: *Studies in anaesthetics,* London, 1967, Lloyd-Luke.

48. Allen, G. D. Minor anesthesia-Chalmers J. Lyons Memorial Lecture, *J Oral Surg* 31:330-335, 1973.

49. Quinn TW, Kendrick TP, Pfeffer RC: The surgical anesthesia team. Symposium on anesthesia and analgesia, *Dent Clin North Am* 17(2):291-304, 1973.

50. Forsyth WD, Allen JD, Everett JB: An evaluation of cardiorespiratory effects of posture in the dental outpatient, *Oral Surg Oral Med Oral Pathol* 34(4):562-580, 1972.

51. Driscoll EJ: Anesthesia morbidity and mortality in oral surgery. Anesthesia for the Ambulatory Patient. Chicago: American Society of Oral Surgeons, September 1966.

52. Lytle JJ: Anesthesia morbidity and mortality survey of the Southern California Society of Oral Surgeons, *J Oral Surg* 32:739, 744, 1974.

53. Lytle JJ, Yoon C: 1978 anesthesia morbidity and mortality survey: Southern California Society of Oral and Maxillofacial Surgeons, *J Oral Surg* 38:814-819, 1980.

54. Campbell RL et al: Respiratory of effects of fentanyl, diazepam, and methohexital sedation, *J Oral Surg* 37:555-562, 1979.

55. Greenblatt DJ, Shader RI: Drug therapy—anticholinergics, *New Engl J Med* 288(23):1215-1218, 1973.

56. Shutt LE, Bowes JB: Atropine and hyocine, *Anaesthesiology* 34:476-490, 1979.

57. Steward DJ, Creighton RE: *General anesthesia for minor surgery in healthy children.* In Gallagher TJ, editor: *Advances in anesthesia,* Chicago, 1984, Year Book.

58. Lavis DM, Lunn JN, Roen M: Glycopyrrolate in children. A comparison between the effects of glycopyrrolate and atropine before induction of anesthesia, *Anaesthesiology* 35:1068-1071, 1981.

59. Drummond-Jackson SL: *Dental sedation and anaesthesia,* ed 6, Oxford, 1979, Society for the Advancement of Anaesthesia in Dentistry.

60. Newman MG et al: A comparative study of psychomotor effects of intravenous agents used in dentistry, *Oral Surg Oral Med Oral Pathol* 30(1):34-40, 1970.

61. Geller E et al: The use of RO 15-1799: a benzodiazepine antagonist in the diagnosis and treatment of benzodiazepine overdose, *Anesthesiology* 61(3A):A135, 1984.

62. Dundee JW, Clarke RSJ: *Noninhalational anesthestics.* In Gray TC et al, editors: *General anaesthesia,* ed 4, London, 1980, Butterworth.

63. White PF: *Anesthesia for ambulatory surgery.* In Stoelting RK et al, editors: *Advanced in anesthesia,* vol 2, Chicago, 1985, Year Book.

64. Wagner RL, White PF: Etomidate vs thiopental—comparative effects on adrenocortical function, *Anesthesiology* 61(A):A353, 1984.

65. Choi SD et al: Comparison of the ventilatory effects of etomidate and methohexital, *Anesthesiology* 62:442-447, 1985.

66. White PF, Way WL, Trevor AJ: Ketamine:its pharmacology and therapeutic uses, *Anesthesiology* 56:119-139, 1982.

67. Becsey L et al: Reduction of the psychomimetic and circulatory side effects of ketamine by droperidol, *Anesthesiology* 37:536-542, 1972.

68. McLaughlin DF, Corcoran RF: Ketamine anesthesia—second thoughts, *Anesth Prog* 20(2):43-45, 1973.

69. Greenfield W: Neuroleptanalgesia, *Dent Clin North Am* 17(2):263-274, 1973.

70. Nagashima H: Personal communication, 1973.

71. Krantz EM: Low-dose intramuscular ketamine and hyaluronidase for induction of anesthesia in non-premedicated children, S. A. Med. Tydsk. 58:161-162, 1980.

72. Yelderman M, New W Jr: Evaluation of pulse oximetry, *Anesthesiology* 59(4):349-352, 1983.

73. Swerdlow DB, Stern S: Continuous noninvasive oxygen saturation monitoring in children with a new pulse oximeter, *Crit Care Med* 228, 1983.

74. Delo RI, Mulkey TF, Davis WH: Monitoring during outpatient anesthesia. Symposium on anesthesia and analgesia, *Dent Clin North Am* 17(2):275-290, 1973.

75. Clark DL, Rosner BS: Neurophysiologic effects of general anesthetics. I. The electroencephalogram and sensory evoked responses in man, *Anesthesiology* 38(6):564-682, 1973.

76. Rosner BS, Clark DL: Neurophysiologic effects of general anesthetics. II. Sequential regional action in the brain, *Anesthesiology* 39(1):59-81, 1973.

77. Zuniga JR: Evidence of central B-endorphin release and recovery after exposure to nitrous oxide (abstract). Washington, DC, October 1985, American Association of Oral Maxillofacial Surgeons.

78. Foldes FF et al: A rational approach to neuroleptanalgesia, *Anesth Anal* 45:642, 1966.

79. Kayama Y, Iwamma K: The EEG, evoked potentials, and single-unity activity during ketamine anesthesia in cats, *Anesthesiology* 36(4):316-328, 1972.

80. Kallar SK, Keenan RL: Evaluation and comparison of recovery time from alfentanil and fentanyl for short surgical procedures, *Anesthesiology* 61 (3A): A379, 1984.

81. MacDonald AG: *The gastric acid problem.* In Atkinson RS et al, editors: *Recent advances in anaesthesia and analgesia,* New York, 1985, Churchill Livingstone.

82. Goudsouzian N et al: Dose-response effects of oral cimetidine on gastric pH and volume in children, *Anesthesiology* 55:533-536, 1981.

83. Somori GJ, Kallar SK, Keenan RL: The effect of cimetidine on gastric pH volume in pediatric patients in an ambulatory surgical center, *Anesthesiology* 61(3A):A448, 1984.

84. Kalb ME, Horne ML, Martz R: Dantrolene in human malignant hyperthermia: multicenter study, *Anesthesiology* 56:254-252, 1982.

85. Schwartz L, Koka BV, Rockoff MA: Masseter spasm after halothane and succinylcholine: incidence and implications, *Anesthesiology* 59(3):A438, 1983.

86. Larach MG, Rosenberg H: Evaluation and management of pediatric patients for diagnostic muscle biopsy for malignant hyperthermia susceptibility, *Anesthesiology* 59(3):A228, 1983.

87. Ellis FR, Heffron JJA: *Clinical and biochemical aspects of malignant hyperypyrexia.* In Atkinson RS et al, editors: *Recent advances in anaesthesia and analgesia,* New York, 1985, Churchill Livingstone.

88. Marx GF, Mateo CV, Orkin LR: Computer analysis of postanesthetic deaths, *Anesthesiology* 39(1):54-58, 1973.

89. Rashad KF et al: Baltimore anesthesia committee: factors in geriatric anesthesia mortality, *Anesth Analg* 44(4):462-468, 1965.

90. Lewin I et al: Physical class and physiologic status in prediction of operative mortality in aged sick, *Ann Surg* 174:217-231, 1971.

91. Vandam LD: Aspiration of gastric contents in the operative period, *N Engl J Med* 273(22):1206-1208, 1965.

92. Mauney FM Jr, Ebert PA, Sabiston DC Jr: Postoperative myocardial infarction: a study of predisposing factors—diagnosis and mortality in a high-risk group of surgical patients, *Ann Surg* 172:497-503, 1970.

93. Miller DH: Medical evaluation of patients with ischemic heart disease prior to anesthesia, *Anesth Prog* 18(2):29-31, 1970.

94. Vaughan RW, et al: Predicting adverse outcomes during anesthesia and surgery by prospective risk assessment, *Anesthesiology* 59(3):A132, 1983.

95. Wilson ME: Morbidity and mortality in anaesthetic practice. In Atkinson RS et al, eds: *Recent advances in anaesthesia and analgesia*, New York, 1985, Churchill Livingstone.

96. Lytle JJ, Stamper EP: The 1988 anesthesia survey of the Southern California Society of Oral and Maxillofacial Surgeons, *J Oral Maxillofac Surg* 47:834-842, 1989.

9

Complications from Anesthesia: Emergencies and Resuscitation

(hasten)

(no response to
painful stimulus?)

(diagnosis of cardio-
respiratory collapse)

(ventilation and
closed-chest cardiac
massage)

(persistence of resusci-
tative efforts brings
favorable results)

29. Then he said to Gehazi,
    gird up thy loins and take
    my staff in thine hand, and
    go thy way: if thou meet
    any man, salute him not;
    and if any salute thee,
    answer him not again: and
    lay my staff upon the face
    of the child.
31. And Gehazi passed on before
    them, and laid the staff
    upon the face of the child;
    but there was neither sound
    nor sign of life. . .
32. And when Elisha was come
    into the house, behold the
    child was dead and laid
    upon his bed.
34. And he went up, and
    lay upon the child, and
    put his mouth upon his
    mouth, and his eyes upon
    his eyes and his hands upon
    his hands; and he stretched
    himself upon the child: and
    the flesh of the child
    waxed warm.
35. Then he returned, and
    walked in the house to and
    fro; and went up, and
    stretched himself upon him:
    and the child sneezed seven
    times and the child opened
    his eyes.

II Kings 4

This biblical recounting of successful cardiopulmonary resuscitation serves as a touchstone for our discussion of complications related to sedation and anesthesia. Specific problems have already been presented in the chapters on local anesthesia, inhalation and intravenous sedation, and, to some extent, general anesthesia. Complications related to general anesthesia are further discussed below, along with recommendations for their prevention and treatment.

Laryngospasm and Airway Obstruction

Preservation of the airway and avoidance of hypoxia are highly important conditions for safe anesthesia practice. Because dentists works in the airway, they must be ever mindful of the potential hazards of obstruction. Such obstruction is most likely to occur at the level of the vocal cords in the hypopharynx. A painful stimulus during anesthetic induction or any foreign material—blood, saliva, tooth fragments, sponges, cotton rolls, etc.—may block the airway and precipitate a spasm of the cords. An attentive assistant with high-flow suction, and the availability of a laryngoscope and Magill forceps for the anesthesia-trained operator, will help to retrieve foreign objects from the throat.

If this condition is compounded by the prior administration of intravenous narcotics and sedatives, then the respiratory center in the medulla is depressed and the hazard is greater. Fortunately, the depressant drug is rapidly redistributed, and if the pharynx is cleared the problem may be easily reversed. The patient should be suctioned and the airway cleared and then a full face mask applied and ventilation assisted with 100% oxygen. It is important to hyperextend the head and neck or move the mandible forward by crooking the fingers behind the mandibular rami to clear the tongue and ensure that the chest rises with each compression of the anesthesia bag.

Allen warns, "Never place anterior traction on the tongue to break laryngeal spasm." He believes that stimulation of the ninth and tenth cranial nerves by this maneuver may precipitate a reflex cardiac arrest.[1] It is rarely necessary to intubate such a patient, although intubation is sometimes required if repeated attempts to continue work are met with repeated spasms. The patient is oxygenated and then given a 40- to 80-mg dose of succinylcholine chloride intravenously, and, with the aid of a laryngoscope, an endotracheal tube is passed and a patent airway ensured.

When someone not trained in intubation techniques is confronted with an obtunded patient with upper airway obstruction, bypassing the blockage at the vocal cord level is imperative. Saliva, blood, and foreign objects in the airway provoke laryngospasm and obstruction. The patient cannot inspire, cough, and eject the obstructing foreign body. Before one proceeds to cricothyrotomy, three maneuvers should be attempted, in rapid succession: (1) suctioning the pharynx with a high-pressure (surgical) suction; (2) administering two to four blows on the back; and (3) performing the Heimlich maneuver—applying forceful compression below the xiphoid process to push residual air in the stomach and lungs upward to "pop the cork" and free the airway. If these three procedures are unsuccessful, there remains one other method—finger probe. This is done to retrieve the foreign body or push it downward, with the option of obstructing one bronchus but allowing the patient to inspire air into the other lung. Vigorous coughing and production of copious secretion often follow. If the foreign object cannot be expelled, a bronchoscopy will be urgently required to remove it from the right lung.

It may be necessary to provide an opening into the trachea below the level of the vocal cords. The procedure of choice is a cricothyrotomy (Fig. 9-1), done with a scalpel blade, a cricothyrotomy needle (Figs. 9-2 to 9-4), or a 14-gauge needle (Fig. 9-5). The use of a sheathed needle ("intracath" or "angiocath") allows perforation with the sharp needle and then cannulation of the trachea by advancing the plastic sheath and removing the metal needle.

The landmarks are easy to identify. With a finger on the thyroid cartilage ("Adam's apple"), slide downward until the depression between the thyroid and cricoid cartilages is felt.

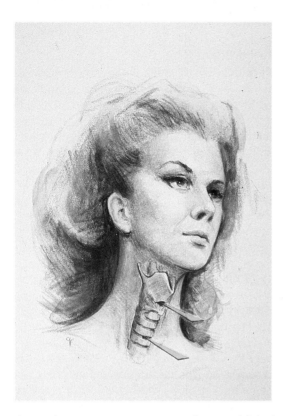

Fig. 9-1. An emergency airway is best established through the cricothyroid membrane (*upper arrow*).

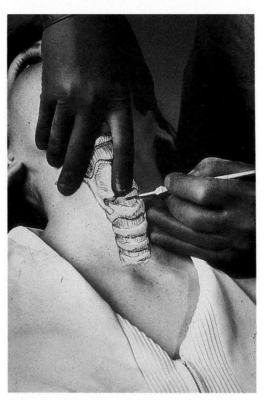

Fig. 9-2. With a finger on the thyroid cartilage a small horizontal incision is made in the depression between the thyroid and cricoid cartilages.

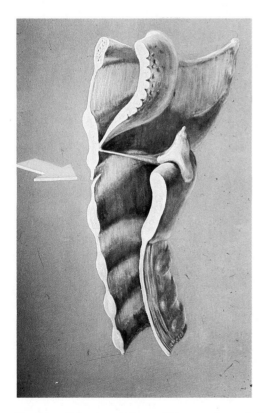

Fig. 9-3. Cricothyrotomy provides an airway below the vocal cords. The thick posterior cricoid cartilage plate helps to minimize the likelihood of a perforation of the posterior wall.

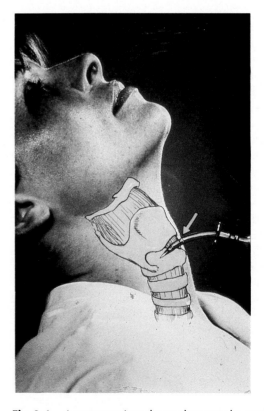

Fig. 9-4. A puncture into the trachea may be made with an Abelson's needle (cricothyrotomy needle) or a 14-gauge needle.

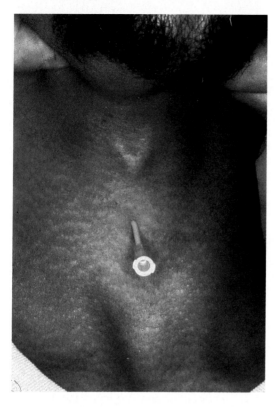

Fig. 9-5. Plastic cannula (14-gauge) in place, bypassing laryngeal obstruction.

Here there are no major vessels and the airway is immediately beneath the skin and fascia, covered only by the cricothyroid membrane. Once the airway is incised or pierced, oxygen is administered directly and the obstructed vocal cords are bypassed. Oxygenation can be maintained by this technique for 30 minutes or longer, until endotracheal intubation is effected.

Although not an emergency procedure, a tracheostomy is fraught with a number of hazards and complications even in the best of hands and circumstances. Experienced surgeons in a well-equipped operating room with good assistants have been known to encounter serious difficulties when doing tracheostomies. In an acute emergency an airway must be established within a very few minutes and the cricothyrotomy is preferred.

Bronchospasm

Respiratory difficulties caused by bronchiolar spasm present as audible wheezing and difficulty in exchanging air. The anesthetist encounters significant resistance in trying to squeeze the bag and inflate the lungs. This condition is analogous to an asthmatic attack and may require that the procedure and anesthesia be stopped if the spasm cannot be overcome. Isoproterenol hydrochloride (Isuprel) or epinephrine may be required to control the spasm. Aminophylline (250 mg) may be given very slowly over a period of 2 to 4 minutes to help relieve the bronchospasm. (Isoproterenol 1 mg is added to 250 ml of 5% dextrose and water and given at a rate of 40 to 60 drops per minute. Alternatively, one or two "puffs" of an Isuprel inhaler may be helpful.)

Epinephrine 0.2 mg may be given subcutaneously, or the "wet-syringe" method may be used for intravenous administration. Here, epinephrine 1:1000 is drawn up into a small syringe (2.5 to 3.0 ml), and then completely expressed back into the epinephrine vial. The residual amount left in the syringe is diluted with the existing saline or dextrose and water being used as the intravenous drip, and then slowly pushed into the running line. Caution is exercised in the use of these agents, especially if the patient has been developing difficulty for a while and has become hypoxic and hypercapnic. In this circumstance, cardiac dysrhythmias are possible.

Cardiac Dysrhythmias

Hypoxia is a primary cause of myocardial irritability and subsequent alterations in heart rate and rhythm. One of the earliest changes in response to hypoxia is an increase in heart rate and the development of tachycardia (rate greater than 100 to 120 beats per minute). Tachycardia may also be initiated by hypercapnia, painful stimulation, and anesthetic drugs. The halogenated anesthetics, such as halothane, methoxyflurane, enflurane, and isoflurane, all sensitize the heart to epinephrine, and caution is urged in the use of local anesthesia containing epinephrine while the patient is receiving these inhalational anesthetics. Anticholinergic drugs such as atropine may produce a tachycardia and, when used with halothane, may produce cardiac dysrhythmias.[1]

Bradycardia (pulse rate less than 60 beats per minute) is usually associated with excessive vagal stimulation, with medications such as the cardiac glycosides (digoxin, digitalis), which induce varying degrees of heart block), or with beta adrenergic blocking agents (e.g., propranolol) which decrease response to epinephrine. The vagus nerve may be stimulated during tracheal intubation, with pressure on the carotid sinus in the neck, or by syncope. Bradycardia is usually treated with the administration of atropine to diminish vagal influence.

A variety of dysrhythmias are seen during anesthesia when the patient is monitored electronically. It has been shown that such continuous careful monitoring will exhibit similar alterations in cardiac rhythm even when a healthy patient is not under the influence of anesthesia. Noble found that almost every cardiac irregularity encountered during general anesthesia was also observed in patients receiving only local anesthesia.[5] Driscoll et al, evaluating the effects of diazepam sedation with local anesthesia, reported a 45% incidence of cardiac dysrhythmias in their local anesthesia control group (mean age, 42 years).[6] The overall incidence of premature ventricular contractions (PVCs) was 3.2% of those patients who showed various dysrhythmias.

Ryder reported a 29% incidence of ectopic ventricular beats in healthy patients undergoing general anesthesia for dental surgery.[7] This was compared with a 9% incidence for those receiving local anesthesia only. The incidence of dysrhythmias was even higher in the older age group. Atropine made no difference in the incidence of dysrhythmias in Ryder's study. He also was able to correlate the onset of dysrhythmias with painful stimulation caused by extraction of teeth and also found that local anesthesia helped to prevent cardiac dysrhythmias.

An occasional PVC has little significance. PVCs do produce a compensatory pause before the next systolic contraction and give an irregular pulse. When PVCs occur more frequently or are multifocal in origin, this usually indicates myocardial irritability of a significant degree and specific measures should be taken immediately. The patient's anesthetic concentration is reduced quickly, and 100% oxygen is given. The surgical procedure should halt until the patient stabilizes. With persistence of the abnormal PVCs an intravenous injection of lidocaine hydrochloride (50 to 100 mg) is given to decrease cardiac irritability. The concern with persisting irritability is the likelihood of its progression to the development of ventricular fibrillation. With fibrillation the heart is functionally inadequate and cardiac output ceases.

Cardiopulmonary Resuscitation

The diagnosis of cardiac "arrest," whether due to fibrillation or asystole, is made on the basis of several important physical signs:

1. Pulse and audible heart sounds and respiration are absent.
2. Skin color becomes dusky gray; blood in the wound becomes dark.
3. Pupils are dilated.
4. Muscles become flaccid.
5. Blood pressure is unobtainable.

Treatment must be instituted immediately if irreversible damage to the central nervous system (CNS) is to be minimized.

Resuscitative efforts are best done by more than one person. Each office should have a well-rehearsed plan of action such that each individual is familiar with his or her responsibilities. (The doctor is the one who spends most time in the office and who is approaching the age when coronary occlusions or sudden life-threatening dysrhythmias can manifest themselves. A doctor's own life may be saved by office assistants who know exactly what to do in the event of a sudden catastrophe.)

The first action should be to initiate ventilation of the lungs. This can be accomplished most directly by the mouth-to-mouth technique (Fig. 9-6). The patient's nostrils are blocked off, and the operator hyperextends the neck to move the tongue away from the oropharynx and prevent obstruction of the airway. In some pa-

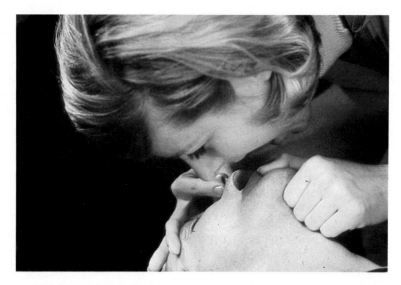

Fig. 9-6. Mouth-to-mouth ventilation with elevation of the chin.

tients, chin lift and jaw thrust forward provide an even better airway than neck hyperextension. Blowing expired air from the operator's lungs should be accompanied by visible expansion of the patient's chest. Another member of the office team provides a firm surface behind the patient's back, usually by placing a board or moving the patient out of the dental chair and onto the floor. This latter maneuver may place the members of the team at a disadvantage when resuscitative efforts are continued over a long period of time. In trying to reach the patient with oxygen via an anesthetic machine, you may find the tubing too short. It is best to be prepared with a firm board to position behind the patient and be able to keep him or her at a better working level.

A full face mask is applied and the patient is ventilated with 100% oxygen by compressing the reservoir bag. Where an anesthesia machine is not immediately available, a self-inflating reservoir bag with or without oxygen attached may be used to ventilate the patient (Fig. 9-7). A manually triggered oxygen-powered ventilation unit is also available (Elder valve, Fig. 9-8), which can readily deliver adequate tidal volumes (500 to 1000 ml per breath).

Mouth-to-mouth ventilation, properly done, is widely recognized as an acceptable and effective method.[8,9] Problems may arise if the stomach is inadvertently expanded with air and vomiting occurs or if the ventilation is much too forceful, especially in young children, and lung tissues are damaged. An unusual complication reported[10] was primary cutaneous tuberculosis resulting from mouth-to-mouth respiration by a medical intern who attempted to resuscitate a patient with fulminant pulmonary tuberculosis.

Cardiac compression is accomplished by depressing the lower end of the sternum in an attempt to squeeze the heart against the vertebrae. With the heel of one hand placed over the lower sternum and with the second hand on top of the first, a forceful thrust is made (Figs. 9-9 and 9-10). These compressions are usually repeated five times, and then a pause is allowed for the ventilator to deliver two breaths. Overall, one attempts to achieve approximately 60 compressions or more per minute. A systolic pressure of 60 to 100 mm Hg can be achieved if the sternum is depressed 3 to 5 cm.[9]

Complications of external cardiac compression include puncture of a lung, rib fracture, or laceration of viscera. Effectiveness of resuscita-

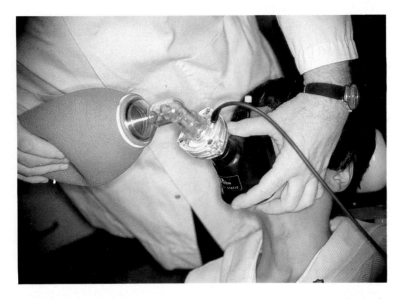

Fig. 9-7. Assisting ventilation with face mask and self-inflating bag. The chin is elevated.

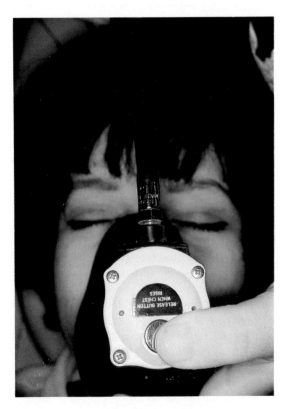

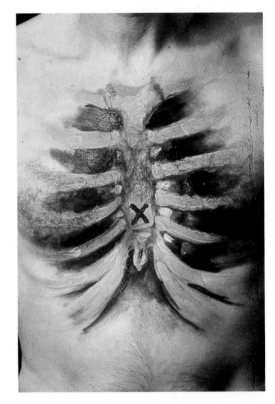

Fig. 9-8. Manually triggered ventilation using the El-der valve—no bag required.

Fig. 9-9. Closed chest compression is directed to the lower end of the sternum.

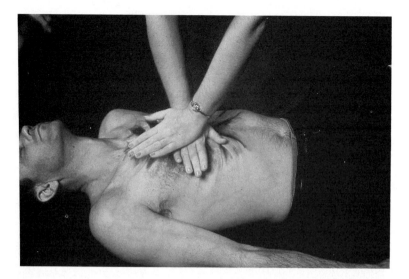

Fig. 9-10.   With the patient on a firm surface, the position of the hands is demonstrated.

tion may be assessed by physical signs of tissue perfusion. For example, if the brain is being oxygenated, the pupils should constrict from their previously dilated condition. Peripheral pulses such as the carotids and femorals may be felt with each cardiac compression, and the patient's skin color should improve.

Other measures designed to enhance the resuscitative effort include endotracheal intubation by an experienced anesthetist to improve ventilation and the addition of drugs (see Fig. 9-9). An intravenous infusion is begun. Sodium bicarbonate is no longer recommended to counter the effects of metabolic acidosis caused by the lack of adequate tissue perfusion by oxygenated blood. Better ventilatory exchange is preferred to drive off carbon dioxide. Other drugs used are atropine sulfate, 0.6 to 1.0 mg given intravenously, and isoproterenol for bradycardia resistant to atropine. Epinephrine (1:1000) is diluted 10 times with sterile water and administered in a 1:10,000 concentration into the running intravenous infusion.

Definitive diagnosis requires the use of an electrocardiograph. If the record shows ventricular fibrillation, a defibrillator is used to shock the heart. If more effective heart function is not achieved immediately, cardiac compression and pulmonary ventilation are continued and a charge of direct current at 200 to 360 joules is tried again. A large number of oral surgeons in the United States are now equipped with cardiac monitors and defibrillators and are trained to provide rapid evaluation and treatment for cardiopulmonary catastrophes.

In the absence of sophisticated equipment, any practitioner can be trained to recognize the problem and institute effective first aid in the form of ventilation and cardiac compression if the need arises. The office staff must be well trained to anticipate this potential problem regardless of whether general anesthetics are used. Each year there is a small but significant number of patients who succumb in dentists' offices, some because of adverse drug reactions and some from natural causes. Many of these patients are eminently resuscitatable (Fig. 9-11).

Approximately 1.5 million acute myocardial infarctions occur in the United States each year, resulting in 528,000 deaths. The survival rate following cardiac arrest secondary to acute myocardial infarction is approximately 10% to 25%. This rises to 50% survival when the patient arrests in a coronary care unit. In the op-

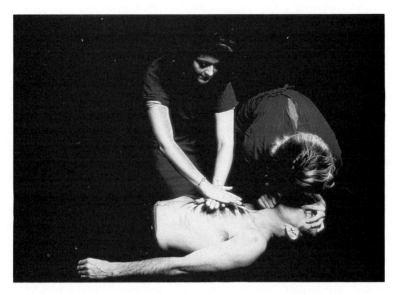

Fig. 9-11. Teamwork is essential for coordinated cardiopulmonary resuscitation.

erating room, success is greater than 50%. In cardiac catheterization laboratories, where patients are monitored constantly, the survival rate reaches 90% or more!

The key is accurate monitoring and immediate cardiopulmonary resuscitation. This must be done by anyone who comes into contact with patients.[9] Many dental schools now include cardiopulmonary resuscitation in their curricula. Some have effectively made it part of their basic science program in physiology and anatomy.

In communities with large numbers of lay persons trained in basic life support (BLS) and with a rapid-response system of well-trained paramedical personnel, resuscitation was successful in more than 40% of patients with documented ventricular fibrillation out of hospital.[9]

Almost all pediatric arrests are secondary to hypoxia. Hyperextension is not recommended; rather a "sniffing" position with mild extension is preferred. Oxygen is given first, then epinephrine and atropine.

Anaphylactic Reaction

Patients who are sensitive to certain drugs may develop a very severe reaction that within min-

utes may lead to urticaria, difficulty in breathing, and cardiovascular collapse. Fortunately its occurrence with local anesthetics and general anesthetics such as the barbiturates is rare.[11] Penicillin, whether taken by mouth or by injection, is responsible for 300 to 1000 deaths in the United States each year.[12,13] This acute antigen-antibody reaction provokes the release of chemical mediators—histamine, slow-reacting substance of anaphylaxis (SRS-A), and eosinophil chemotactic factor of anaphylaxis (ECF-A), which act to increase vascular permeability, contract smooth muscle, and attract inflammatory cells.[14]

Atopic patients with a prior history of symptoms on exposure to an allergen and with a family history of similar reactions are particularly susceptible. Antihistamines are *not* effective in the management of this type of overwhelming reaction. Epinephrine 1:1000, 0.3 to 0.5 mg, is given subcutaneously to abort the attack. It may have to be repeated. A comparison of intralingual and intravenous epinephrine before and during anaphylactic shock and cardiac depression showed that the intralingual route was much less effective than the intravenous route. Both the onset of action and the blood levels achieved by the intralingual route were such as to question their use and efficacy in resuscitative efforts.[15] Additional supportive therapy includes the administration of oxygen and the addition of corticosteroids in large doses (e.g., hydrocortisone 100 to 500 mg intravenously).

Intra-Arterial Injection

A few simple precautions are taken to avoid intra-arterial injection. The area is first palpated for any pulsations. In the antecubital fossa, 15% to 18% of patients have a superficial branch of the brachial artery.[1] This is more often the case on the medial aspect of the fossa, where the ulnar artery may course superficial to the biceps aponeurosis, when the brachial artery branches higher up in the arm. Palpation should be done prior to placing the tourniquet, which may dampen or even block the pulsations of the smaller arteries if it is applied too tightly. Although the dorsum of the hand has been suggested as a "safe" area, reports of intra-arterial pentothal involving this approach have also been reported.[16]

With the use of a continuous saline infusion technique, intra-arterial injection can be avoided. Entry into an artery causes more pain than venipuncture, and the infusion of any solution is experienced as pain more peripheral to the site of injection. If saline alone is infused, no complications will result.

It may be difficult to run the infusion into an artery, against the systolic pressure gradient. The drip will be very slow or will not run at all. Blood of brighter color may be seen to pulsate back into the capillary tube extension of the needle. The technique of an indwelling needle attached to a benign infusion solution offers many more safeguards than the "hit-and-run" tactic of injecting a syringe full of medication and then withdrawing the needle. Even if the needle is not withdrawn and is allowed to sit in the vessel, it will frequently plug up. No medication need ever be injected until the operator confirms that the needle is properly positioned in a vein.

Intra-arterial injection leading to a necrosis and gangrene of digits has been reported to oc-

cur by self-administration in drug addicts.[17] It has also been reported after infusion of thiopental and methohexital, especially with more concentrated solutions than those usually given. The damage is not the result of the short-lived arterial spasm but is due to crystal formation, endothelial damage, and subsequent thrombosis of the artery.[18,19] Efforts to treat the injury are directed toward early heparinization of the patient to inhibit clot formation, or the early introduction of thrombolytic agents such as tPA, streptokinase, or urokinase. Injury has been directly related to the concentration of the barbiturate, and it is recommended that concentration of thiopental not exceed 2.5% and that methohexital not exceed 1%. The injection of procaine to produce vasodilation or even a local anesthetic block of the sympathetic ganglion is of very limited value because of the transient effects of either.

Summary

Serious complications may attend general anesthesia: of crucial concern is the integrity of a patent airway. Efforts to maintain good ventilatory exchange may be compromised by the development of a laryngospasm. Fortunately, once the oropharynx has been cleared and suctioned, the administration of 100% oxygen by full face mask usually restores ventilation to normal. Failure to achieve reversal of laryngospasm would indicate an emergent need for either tracheal intubation or cricothyrotomy to bypass the blocked vocal cords and re-establish respiratory exchange.

Hypoxia develops rapidly and sensitizes the heart to the development of cardiac dysrhythmias. Premature ventricular contractions that occur with increasing frequency may herald the development of ventricular tachycardia and ventricular fibrillation. Efforts are directed to improve the patient's oxygenation and defer further painful manipulations until the cardiac status improves and stabilizes.

Recognition of the early signs of cardiac arrest are necessary to be able to put into effect the proper resuscitative measures. Delay defines disaster. Each individual in the office should know exactly what his or her role is in the resuscitative effort.

Ventilation is first re-established either by the mouth-to-mouth method or by anesthetic reservoir bag with adjunctive oxygen. Intubation may be delayed, particularly if ventilation by other techniques is effective in raising the chest with each respiration. Closed chest compressions at approximately 60 or more times per minute are begun in an effort to rhythmically squeeze the heart between the depressed sternum and the vertebrae. Additional supportive measures include the intravenous administration of drugs such as atropine, epinephrine, and others. Electrical defibrillation is applied once the diagnosis has been established. Successful cardiopulmonary resuscitation is largely dependent upon the ability of those around the patient to recognize the problem and render immediate care.

Intra-arterial anesthetic injections are preventable. Nevertheless, inadvertent arterial injections have been a primary cause of digital necrosis, especially when highly concentrated anesthetic solutions are used. They cause endothelial damage with subsequent clot formation, leading to thrombosis of the involved artery and consequent ischemia of tissues. Early treatment is aimed at heparinization or thrombolytic therapy to enhance continued perfusion of the limb.

A knowledge of the potential complications serves to alert one to the need for specific preventive measures as well as remedial procedures.

References

1. Allen GD: *Dental anesthesia and analgesia,* 3, Baltimore, 1984, William & Wilkins.
2. Jacoby JJ et al: Transtracheal resuscitation, *J Am Med Assoc* 162(7):625-628, 1956.
3. Cosgriff JH Jr: *An atlas of diagnostic and therapeutic procedures for emergency personnel,* Philadelphia, 1978, JB Lippincott.
4. Attia RR, Baittit GE, Murphy JD: Transtracheal ventilation, *J Am Med Assoc* 162(7):625-628, 1956.
5. Noble FP: Electrocardiographic findings during out-patient anesthesia, *Anesth Prog* 16(5):161-171, 1969.
6. Driscoll EJ et al: Sedation with intravenous diazepam, *J Oral Surg* 30:332-343, 1972.
7. Ryder W: The electrocardiogram in dental anesthesia, *Anesthesiology* 25(1):46-62, 1970.
8. McIntyre KN, Parker MR: 1979 National Conference on Cardiopulmonary Resuscitation and Emergency Cardiac Care, *J Am Med Assoc* 244(5):453-509, 1980.
9. Donegan J: New concepts in CPR, *Anesth Prog* 27(4):121-124, 1980.
10. Heilmann KM, Muschenheim C: Primary cutaneous tuberculosis resulting from mouth-to-mouth respiration, *N Engl J Med* 273(19):1035-1036, 1965.
11. Holmes RP, Ross JW, Williams ER: Acute anaphylaxis under anesthesia, *Anesthesiology* 26(3):363-367, 1971.
12. Krapin D: Anaphylaxis with orally administered penicillin, *N Engl J Med* 267:820, 1962.
13. Stewart G, and McGovern J: *Penicillin allergy: clinical and immunologic aspects (II),* Springfield, Ill, 1970, Charles C Thomas.
14. Austen KF: Systemic anaphylaxis in the human being, *N Engl J Med* 291(13):661-664, 1974.
15. Halperin SD, Hunt LM, Yagiela JA: A comparison of intralingual and intravenous epinephrine before and during cardiovascular depression, *Oral Surg Oral Med Oral Pathol* 46(3):333-343, 1978.
16. Lynes RFA, Bisset WIK: Intra-arterial thiopentone: inadvertent injection through a cannula on the back of the hand, *Anesthesiology* 24(2):257-261, 1969.
17. Topazian RG: Accidental intra-arterial injection: a hazard of intravenous medication, *J Am Dent Assoc* 81(2):410-416, 1970.
18. Waters DJ: Intra-arterial thiopentone: a physico-chemical phenomenon, *Anesthesiology* 21(3):346-356, 1966.
19. Brown SS, Lyons SM, Dundee JW: Intra-arterial barbiturates, *Br J Anaesth* 40(13):13-19, 1968.
20. *Textbook of advanced cardiac life support* ed 2, 1987, American Heart Association.

10

Postoperative Pain Control

A broad spectrum of measures for the management of postoperative pain is in keeping with the overall philosophy of pain control proposed by this book. Just as there is no one method that can provide universally satisfactory relief of operative anxiety and pain, so there is no postoperative panacea. Instead, each individual may require special instruction and treatment. However, there are certain generalizations that may be drawn to support postoperative care.

It has been repeatedly demonstrated that better informed patients can better handle their postoperative reactions. A patient who knows what to expect by way of swelling, bleeding, and discomfort after surgical treatment can be prepared and will respond with less fear and anxiety. Egbert et al have shown the importance of preoperative orientation to postsurgical behavior.[1,2] When compared with controls, their "special-care" patients who had been instructed preoperatively requested only half as much narcotic medication after surgery, were ready for earlier discharge from the hospital, and had an overall better recovery. It is important to advise an oral surgical patient realistically during the consultation visit about his or her postoperative course, including when and for how long pain may be anticipated. This is repeated when instructions are given after surgery.

Specifically, postoperative pain may be severe for 8 to 12 hours after the local anesthetic wears off, and the patient should be provided medication for that period. Patients should be further advised that by the following day their pain will abate, although they should expect soreness, which will respond to mild analgesics. In a high percentage of cases, patients returning the following week report this exact sequence. They are thus provided with a "program" and know what to expect, which serves to lessen anxiety. The doctor's home telephone number can be provided in the event a weekend or holiday recess follows surgery. In almost 35 years of a surgical practice, only a small handful of patients have called me—in some cases they were checking to be reassured and did not want me to see them until the day the office was regularly open. Pain worsens when anxiety goes unchecked. Anxiety is reduced by establishing a warm, understanding relationship.

In repeated studies of postoperative dental and jaw pain the therapeutic efficacy of placebos has been supported. In such studies, approximately one third of patients report no pain and find it unnecessary to take any medication. In White's study of postextraction pain, 75% of those patients using placebo tablets reported pain relief.[3]

Frank suggests that the effectiveness of the placebo lies in its ability to mobilize the patient's expectancy of help.[4] Placebo responders tended to be more dependent, emotionally reactive, and conventional, while the nonreactors were more likely to be isolated and mistrustful. He concludes that the ability to respond favorably to a placebo is not so much a sign of excessive gullibility as of easy acceptance of others in their socially defined roles. Lasagna et al found it difficult to readily typify placebo reactors by superficial interviews.[5]

Recently, with an expansion of our knowledge of the neural mechanisms involved in pain transmission, the mode of action of placebos has been re-explored. Levine, Gordon, and Fields reported that the narcotic antagonist naloxone hydrochloride antagonized placebo effects.[6] Gordon showed a variable (biphasic) effect of naloxone on pain, with low dosage being analgesic.[7] Placebo analgesia is thought to be a form of conditioning.[8]

Placebos are increasingly effective under conditions of increased stress. Beecher showed that placebo effectiveness amounted to 77% that of morphine when the pain was the severest.[9]

With such a powerful placebo effect at the doctor's disposal, he or she should make use of its influence. Acute pain following dental and oral surgical manipulations usually runs a predictable course in the absence of infection and complications. The pain is at its peak when the local anesthetic wears off, and it continues at a worrisome and discomforting level for the next 8 to 12 hours. Beyond this time postsurgical pain becomes less acute and gradually fades into a dull soreness.

Protecting against this first painful period may be planned for by requesting that the patient take the medication well before the local anesthetic has worn off so that he or she is not suddenly "hit" by acute pain.

For the patient who reacts adversely to oral or intramuscular analgesics, it may be helpful to use a long-acting regional anesthetic (see Chapter 4).

The use of bupivacaine hydrochloride, a newer local anesthetic that binds readily to protein, provides anesthesia and analgesia that has been shown to last 7 to 12 hours after a nerve block.[10] In addition, it appears that bupivacaine is different from other local anesthetic agents in that the duration of anesthesia is influenced by the dosage given. Dosages of 0.5% (5 mg/ml bupivacaine hydrochloride [Marcaine]), with and without 1:200,000 epinephrine, are available in dental cartridges. Increasing the dosage or using a stronger concentration (0.75% [7.5 mg/ml]) resulted in even longer periods of anesthesia and analgesia.

If the patient is hospitalized and readily available, the doctor may prefer to repeat the regional nerve block to ensure continued analgesia and circumvent the need for systemic analgesics entirely.

Both wine and stronger alcoholic spirits have been used since antiquity to diminish pain. They may be recommended for postoperative pain relief because they possess both sedative and analgesic properties and may be available in the household where other pharmaceutical analgesics are not.

Other measures are useful for control of discomfort. Many patients obtain symptomatic relief from the use of ice packs following surgery. Ethyl chloride spray to the facial skin overlying the masticator muscles has helped to overcome painful postoperative trismus. Local heat applied to these areas also helps to decrease the edema and mobilize sore muscles. Adrenocorticosteroids such as dexamethasone (Decadron) have been used to limit edema and the inflammatory response. The steroid should be given 6 to 12 hours preoperatively and continued for 48 hours for optimal results.

Preliminary studies with a combination of long-acting local anesthetic and dexamethasone and a nonsteroidal anti-inflammatory agent given at the time of surgery significantly reduced the incidence and severity of postsurgical pain and the need for postoperative narcotic analgesics.

The anti-inflammatory agents work by inhibiting the synthesis of prostaglandins and by reducing pain and swelling.[11] They also have some adverse effects, particularly in patients prone to develop gastrointestinal problems. Like acetylsalicylic acid, they interfere with platelet aggregation and may exacerbate coagulopathies or bleeding disorders. They are contraindicated in patients who are allergic to aspirin.

Other local measures include various packs for periodontal surgery and exodontia. The packing of a "dry socket" (alveolar osteitis) is a widespread practice. Each practitioner introduces his or her own particular trusted recipe that forms the basis for the mixture. Basically, the less damaging the dressing, the quicker the recovery, the greater the comfort, and the greater the chances of normal healing. Various escharotic drugs invariably produce more tissue and bone necrosis and lead to protracted healing.

Alveolar osteitis following extraction produces severe pain and a fetid odor usually beginning 48 to 72 hours postoperatively. It is most often associated with mandibular third molar extractions and with traumatic removal of brittle teeth. The incidence of postoperative osteitis sharply increases in smokers (12%) as compared to nonsmokers (2.5%). The delayed onset of symptoms, the lack of overt pus, the fetid odor, as well as lysis and loss of the clot, all suggest that slowly growing anaerobic organisms are producing proteolytic enzymes, endotoxins, and collagenase. Some pathogenic gram-negative anaerobes are not penicillin- or tetracycline-sensitive and may be the cause of alveolar osteitis.

Recent studies have shown the efficacy of the use of a topical antibiotic known to be effective against gram-negative anaerobes. After copious irrigation of the socket with saline, an absorbable gelatin sponge saturated with clindamycin solution is inserted. Within 2 to 4 hours the pain abates and no further dressing changes are required. Double-blind studies of a placebo versus clindamycin have verified the efficacy of clindamycin in preventing "dry sockets" as well as successfully treating them when they develop.[12]

Clinical studies of the efficacy of selected analgesics are subject to a wide variability of patient response. In a triple-blind study of postextraction pain Jacobs et al compared five commonly used analgesic preparations (three of which contained codeine), to codeine phosphate alone and to another control drug containing acetylsalicylic acid, pentobarbital, and three anticholinergic drugs in combination.[13] Results showed these combinations superior to codeine phosphate by itself—even the drug combination without codeine provided more pain relief than codeine alone.

Getter, Levin, and Ayer also compared the effectiveness of some commonly prescribed analgesics and concluded that aspirin by itself provided "almost complete" or "complete" pain relief in over 80% of their subjects; codeine with aspirin provided similar relief in 73% of

their patients; propoxyphene hydrochloride (Darvon) provided 56% relief, and the placebo provided only 12% relief.[14] Of further interest in these studies is the finding that a number of patients who received the experimental medication reported side effects and discontinued the study drug, only to select the identical medication from their own sources and take it without problems.

Procedurally, each patient should be acquainted with the postoperative course to be anticipated: a prescription should be made available to the patient, and the patient should be advised that this medication be taken before the local anesthetic wears off completely. The patient is further advised that the pain will be largely controlled by the medication but not necessarily completely eliminated. The pain will abate after the first 12 hours, and little or no medication will be required the next day and thereafter.

Some of the oldest agents used in the relief of mild to moderate pain are the salicylates. This family of drugs includes acetylsalicylic acid, sodium salicylate, and choline salicylate (Arthropan). The choline form has some advantage in that it does not have the antiplatelet effect seen with acetylsalicylic acid and can be used in patients who have bleeding tendencies.

The mechanism of action of the salicylates relates to their anti-inflammatory effect and to their interaction with prostaglandins. Some other agents classified as nonsteroidal anti-inflammatory (NSAI) analgesics include diflunisal (Dolobid), ibuprofen (Motrin), and naproxen (Naprosyn). Salicylates and the NSAI agents have some unpleasant side effects, principally gastrointestinal irritation (to be avoided in patients with peptic ulcer disease). Dizziness, tinnitus, skin rashes, and rare severe allergic reactions occur with salicylates. Applied topically to oral mucosa the salicylates produce a chemical burn with necrosis and sloughing of tissue and should not be used topically in the mouth. Salicylates are available in 300-mg tablets, and one or two tablets are prescribed to be taken every 3 to 4 hours. No greater analgesic effect is achieved by a dose larger than 600 mg. The recommended dosages of the three NSAI agents mentioned is as follows: diflunisal, 500 to 1000 mg to start and 500 mg every 8 to 12 hours; ibuprofen, 400 mg every 6 to 8 hours; naproxen, 250 to 500 mg twice per day.

Acetaminophen, a major metabolite of phenacetin, has analgesic effects similar to acetylsalicylic acid but has minimal anti-inflammatory effects. It is safe to use in patients with peptic ulcer disease because it does not provoke gastric irritation. It is also recommended over aspirin for asthmatic patients who wheeze when taking aspirin, for patients with coagulation defects, and for patients with gout.[15] Hypersensitivity reactions to acetaminophen are rare and may present as laryngeal edema, skin rash, urticaria, neutropenia, or pancytopenia. Toxic doses lead to hepatic injury and methemoglobinemia. Acetaminophen is prescribed as 300 to 600 mg every 3 to 4 hours. Phenacetin taken in large doses together with other analgesics has been implicated in the causation of renal injury, but the relationship has not been completely defined.

Pentazocine hydrochloride (Talwin), which is a nonopioid agent chemically related to morphine, had been promoted for pain control. It was not subjected to federal narcotic control. Pharmacologically it produces analgesia, acting like a narcotic, although when compared to aspirin it is not significantly different in effect. Some of its more disturbing side effects include dizziness, impaired thinking, and hallucinations. As with narcotics, tolerance occurs as does respiratory depression. Its use in ambulatory patients is limited primarily by its unusual central nervous system effects. It has fallen from favor over the recent past.

Codeine phosphate is the analgesic drug most commonly used along with aspirin (acetylsalicylic acid): 30 to 60 mg every 3 to 4 hours is usually adequate to control mild to moderate pain. One of the problematic side effects of codeine, and indeed all narcotics, is the tendency to cause nausea and vomiting. This is particularly true for ambulatory patients. Although the incidence of nausea and vomiting is also dose related, it may involve almost 30% of patients on moderately low dosage. Codeine also produces some drowsiness. The onset of action, when the drug is taken orally, is approximately 20 to 30 minutes. If 60 mg of codeine is ineffective in relieving pain, larger doses will be of limited value and may cause restlessness and even more dizziness, nausea, and vomiting. If the medication at this dosage level is inadequate, other, stronger agents may be prescribed.

Percodan is a combination of analgesics with approximately 5 mg of oxycodone hydrochloride per tablet instead of codeine. The other ingredients include aspirin, phenacetin, and caffeine. As an analgesic, oxycodone is almost equivalent to morphine in potency, and its addiction liability is also equivalent. With this in mind, it may be used for limited exposure to achieve greater relief of moderately severe pain in the postoperative period.

Percocet contains 5 mg of oxycodone hydrochloride but differs from Percodan in the substitution of acetaminophen for the aspirin, phenacetin, and caffeine. The recommended dose is one to two tablets every 4 to 6 hours, depending on the severity of the pain. Side effects are comparable to Percodan and to codeine, with a possible diminution in the incidence of nausea and vomiting.

Hydromorphone hydrochloride (Dilaudid) is a potent narcotic analgesic that is available for oral ingestion. A dosage of 1 or 2 mg every 3 to 4 hours is equivalent to 5 to 10 mg of morphine. The same side effects as with all narcotics exist: patients experience dizziness, nausea, vomiting, and, with increasing dosage, respiratory depression.

A number of other narcotic analgesics are available. For example, meperidine hydrochloride (Demerol) is widely used. In our experience, for postoperative relief of moderately severe pain, 100 to 150 mg of meperidine hydrochloride is necessary. It offers few if any real advantages over other narcotics.

The narcotic antagonist naloxone hydrochloride (Narcan) is an important agent to effect reversal of narcotic-induced respiratory depression. It is available in a 0.4 mg/ml solution for intravenous, intramuscular, or subcutaneous injection and effectively counteracts all of the narcotic's properties. In the absence of prior narcotics, naloxone is free of side effects. It is not effective against nonopioid drugs such as barbiturates and tranquilizers, nor will it intensify the respiratory depression. Naloxone's effect is short lived when given intravenously and may require repeat dosage.[16]

Attention has been drawn to the occurrence of various birth defects in relation to drugs ingested during pregnancy. The thalidomide tragedy of the early 1960s stimulated clinicians and researchers to study the subject of drug use during pregnancy more closely. A large number of drugs are consumed by pregnant women: the second most common of the drug categories is analgesics. Compounds that are highly lipid soluble, of low molecular weight, and not ionized pass the placenta readily. The placenta also has some limited ability to detoxify and metabolize drugs. Few drugs have been definitely linked to specific birth defects.[17] Most pregnant women, especially during the first trimester, would do well to avoid elective treatment and whatever associated psychic, physical, and pharmacologic stresses it may impose on the developing fetus. Later during pregnancy, elective and urgent dental treatment is generally well tolerated. All medication should be used sparingly and only if required. Other aids and techniques to relieve discomfort, cited earlier in this chapter, may be employed to help avoid systemic medication.

Caution is advised with the administration of postoperative analgesics, especially if the patient is also taking other medications, particularly sedatives, tranquilizers, and CNS depressants. The combined effects of these agents serve to intensify the depressant effects and may lead to hypoventilation, hypoxia, and hypercapnia, with secondary damage to vital organs.

Pain medication should be prescribed in amount and number that will not leave an excess of drug available after the immediate need is over, because this can encourage abuse. Postoperative complications often signal their presence by renewed pain and swelling. Definitive diagnosis and treatment, such as incision and drainage of an abscess plus antibiotic treatment, should be carried out rather than trying to obtund the pain without treatment of the infection.

Summary

Management of postoperative pain requires a flexibility of approaches reminiscent of the total spectrum of pain control recommended for preoperative and intraoperative methods. Underlying this choice of method is the concern for individualizing treatment. A significant number of patients experience no postoperative pain. An even larger group of patients shows dramatic relief of pain in response to placebo medication. At best, the postoperative period of pain is a circumscribed experience that will improve with the passage of time. In the absence of complications, such as infection, postsurgical pain is limited in duration to 8 to 12 hours. Patients should be honestly advised of the anticipated sequence of these postoperative events. It has been shown repeatedly that patients properly informed preoperatively will experience less discomfort, require less pain medication, and have a more successful postoperative course, with earlier recovery and even earlier discharge from the hospital.

Local as well as systemic measures are taken to relieve postoperative discomfort. Systemic analgesics are often used to quell pain and anxiety following surgery. These may be nonnarcotic analgesics such as aspirin, acetaminophen, and nonsteroidal anti-inflammatory agents. Narcotic analgesics may be required for conditions of moderate to severe pain: codeine phosphate, Percodan, Percocet, meperidine hydrochloride (Demerol), and hydromorphone hydrochloride (Dilaudid) constitute a small group of oral analgesics that provide adequate pain relief but also have some disturbing side effects. Dizziness, nausea and vomiting, and constipation attend the use of narcotics, particularly for ambulatory patients. In high dosage, respiratory depression also occurs. Narcotic analgesics also carry the liability for addiction, particularly if used over a longer period of time. This is unusual in dentistry because of the limited nature of the postoperative period, but may become a problem in patients with long-term facial pain.

Caution should attend the administration of any medication during the first trimester of pregnancy. In general, elective treatments should be deferred until the second and third trimesters, and systemic medications should be given only if essential. The coadministration of other sedatives, tranquilizers, and CNS depressants also indicates a need for caution when analgesics are prescribed.

References

1. Egbert LD et al: The value of the preoperative visit by anesthetist: a study of doctor-patient rapport, *JAMA* 185(7):553-555, 1963.
2. Egbert LD et al: Reduction of postoperative pain by encouragement and instruction of patients; a study of doctor-patient rapport, *N Engl J Med* 270(16):825-827, 1964.
3. White WL et al: A comparison of analgesic agents in dentistry, *J Dent Res* 37:13, 1958.
4. Frank JD: *Persuasion and healing:* a comparative study of psychotherapy, Baltimore, 1961, The John Hopkins Press.
5. Lasagna L et al: Study of the placebo response, *Am J Med* 16:770, 1954.
6. Levine JD, Gordon NC, Fields HL: The narcotic antagonist naloxone enhances clinical pain, *Nature (Lond)* 272:826, 1978.
7. Gordon NC: Method of administration determines the effect of naloxone on pain (abstract).
8. Watkins LR, Mayer DJ: Organization of endogenous opiate and nonopiate pain control systems, *Science* 216:1185-1192, 1982.
9. Beecher HK: The powerful placebo, *J Am Med Assoc* 159:1602, 1955.
10. Trieger N, Gillen GH: Bupivacaine anesthesia and postoperative analgesia in oral surgery, *Anesth Prog* 26(1):20-23, 1979.
11. Troullos ES et al: Comparison of nonsteroidal anti-inflammatory drugs, ibuprofen and flurbiprofen, with methylprednisolone and placebo for acute pain, swelling and trismus, *J Oral Maxillofac Surg* 48:945-952, 1990.
12. Trieger N, Schlagel G: Etiology and prevention of alveolar osteitis—"dry socket," *J Am Dent Assoc* 122:67-68, 1991.
13. Jacobs AW et al: A comparative study of 5 analgesic agents, *Anesth Prog* 17:105, 1970.
14. Getter L, Levin MP, Ayer WA: Comparative effectiveness of some commonly prescribed drugs for the relief of postsurgical discomfort, *Anesth Prog* 20:4, 1973.
15. Koch-Weser J: Drug therapy: acetaminophen, *N Engl J Med* 295:1297-1300, 1976.
16. Actkenhead AR et al: Pharmacokinetics of intravenous naloxone in healthy volunteers, *Anesthesiology* 61(3A):A381, 1984.
17. Marx JL: Drugs during pregnancy: do they affect the unborn child? *Science* 180:174-175, 1973.

American Association of Oral Maxillofacial Surgeons, Washington, DC, Oct 1985.

Appendix: Some Trade and Generic Names Used in this Book

Adrenaline (epinephrine chloride): Parke-Davis, Morris Plains, N.J.

Alfenta (alfentanil hydrochloride): Janssen Pharmaceutica, Titusville, N.J.

Atarax (hydroxyzine hydrochloride): Roerig, New York, N.Y.

Benadryl (diphenhydramine hydrochloride): Parke-Davis, Morris Plains, N.J.

Brevital (methohexital sodium): Eli Lilly, Indianapolis, Ind.

Carbocaine (mepivacaine hydrochloride): Eastman Kodak, Rochester, N.Y.

Citanest (prilocaine): Astra Pharmaceutical, Westboro, Mass.

Cleocin (clindamycin phosphate): Upjohn, Kalamazoo, Mich.

Compazine (prochlorperazine maleate): Smith Kline Beecham, Pittsburgh, Pa.

Dantrium (dantrolene sodium): Procter & Gamble, Norwich, N.Y.

Darvon (propoxyphene hydrochloride): Eli Lilly, Indianapolis, Ind.

Decadron (dexamethasone): Merck & Co., West Point, Pa.

Demerol (meperidine hydrochloride): Sanofi Winthrop Pharmaceuticals, New York, N.Y.

Dilaudid (hydromorphone hydrochloride): Knoll, Whippany, N.J.

Diprivan (propofol): Stuart, Wilmington, Del.

Diuril (chlorothiazide): Merck & Co., West Point, Pa.

Dolobid (diflunisal): Merck & Co., West Point, Pa.

Duranest (etidocaine hydrochloride): Astra Pharmaceutical, Westboro, Mass.

Elavil (amitriptyline hydrochloride): Stuart, Wilmington, Del.

Ethrane (enflurane): Anaquest, Liberty Corner, N.J.

Fluothane (halothane): Wyeth-Ayerst, Philadelphia, Pa.

Forane (isoflurane): Anaquest, Liberty Corner, N.J.

Halcion (triazolam): Upjohn, Kalamazoo, Mich.

Haldol (haloperidol): McNeil, Spring House, Pa.

Hydrodiuril (hydrochlorothiazide): Smith Kline Beecham, Pittsburgh, Pa.

Inderal (propranolol hydrochloride): Wyeth-Ayerst, Philadelphia, Pa.

Isoptin (verapamil hydrochloride): Knoll, Whippany, N.J.

Isuprel (isoproterenol hydrochloride): Sanofi Winthrop Pharmaceuticals, New York, N.Y.

Ketalar (ketamine hydrochloride): Park-Davis, Morris Plains, N.J.

Lasix (furosemide): Hoechst-Roussel, Somerville, N.J.

Librium (chlordiazepoxide hydrochloride): Roche, Nutley, N.J.

Marcaine (bupivacaine hydrochloride): Eastman Kodak, Rochester, N.Y.

Mellaril (thioridazine hydrochloride): Sandoz Pharmaceuticals, East Hanover, N.J.

Motrin (ibuprofen): Upjohn, Kalamazoo, Mich.

Naprosyn (naproxen): Syntex, Palo Alto, Calif.

Narcan (naloxone hydrochloride): Astra, Westboro, Mass.

Nembutal (pentobarbital sodium): Abbott, North Chicago, Ill.

Nisentil (alphaprodine hydrochloride): off the market

Penthrane (methoxyflurane): Abbott, North Chicago, Ill.

Pentothal (thiopental): Abbott, North Chicago, Ill.

Percodan (oxycodone hydrochloride): Du Pont Pharmaceuticals, Wilmington, Del.

Percocet (oxycodone and acetaminophen): Du Pont Pharmaceuticals, Wilmington, Del.

Phenergan (promethazine hydrochloride): Wyeth-Ayerst, Philadelphia, Pa.

Procardia (nifedipine): Pfizer, New York, N.Y.

Prozac (fluoxetine hydrochloride): Dista, Indianapolis, Ind.

Robinul (glycopyrrolate): A. H. Robins Co., Richmond, Va.

Seconal (secobarbital sodium): Wyeth-Ayerst, Philadelphia, Pa.

Stadol (butorphanol tartrate): Mead Johnson, Princeton, N.J.

Sublimaze (fentanyl citrate): Janssen Pharmaceutica, Titusville, N.J.

Tagamet (cimetadine): Smith Kline Beecham Pharmaceuticals, Pittsburgh, Pa.

Talwin (pentazocine hydrochloride): Sanofi Winthrop Pharmaceuticals, New York, N.Y.

Thorazine (chlorpromazine hydrochloride): Smith Kline Beecham, Pittsburgh, Pa.

Tofranil (imipramine hydrochloride): Geigy Pharmaceutical, Ardsley, N.Y.

Valium (diazepam): Roche, Nutley, N.J.

Versed (midazolam hydrochloride): Roche, Nutley, N.J.

Vistaril (hydroxyzine hydrochloride): Pfizer, New York, N.Y.

Xylocaine (lidocaine hydrochloride): Astra, Westboro, Mass.

Zantac (ranitidine hydrochloride): Glaxo, Research Triangle Park, N.C.

Index

Page numbers in *italics* indicate illustrations. Page numbers followed by *t* indicate tables.